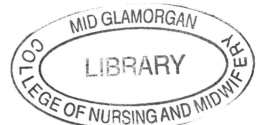

# Preventing Coronary Artery Disease

*Cardioprotective Therapeutics in the 1990s*

# Preventing Coronary Artery Disease

*Cardioprotective Therapeutics in the 1990s*

**Martin J Kendall** MD FRCP

Clinical Pharmacology Section
Department of Medicine
University of Birmingham
Queen Elizabeth Hospital
Birmingham B15 2TH, UK

**Richard C Horton** BSc MB

The Lancet
42 Bedford Square
London WC1B 3SL, UK

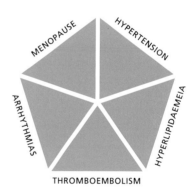

**MARTIN DUNITZ**

First published in the United Kingdom in 1994 by
Martin Dunitz Ltd
The Livery House
7–9 Pratt Street
London NW1 0AE

A CIP catalogue record for this book is available
from the British Library.

ISBN 1-85317-175-1

Composition by Scribe Design, Gillingham, Kent
Printed and bound in Singapore by Kyodo Printing Co (S'pore) Pte Ltd

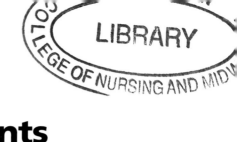

# Contents

Dedicated to

Rosemary

Clarice and Ken

# Preface

As clinicians and writers, we are constantly struck by how few attempts are made both practically and intellectually to integrate the different therapeutic approaches to coronary artery disease (CAD) into a single coherent management programme for the individual patient.

Since in most patients the first major coronary event is sudden death or a silent infarction, mortality rates can only be reduced substantially by prophylactic measures. These include lifestyle changes with advice on smoking cessation in particular but also, for example, on weight, diet and exercise where appropriate. Drug therapy, the subject of this book, should be offered in conjunction with and not instead of these non-pharmacological measures.

Our first aim is to argue that patients at increased risk of a coronary event and who need treatment should be offered drugs that have the potential to reduce that risk. Our emphasis has been on prophylaxis and longer term cardioprotective measures. Our second aim is to propose a broad approach to reducing coronary mortality. Patients may be at increased risk from hypertension, hyperlipidaemia, arrhythmias, thromboembolism and, in the female, the postmenopausal state. The heart can be protected from these five perspectives; yet doctors, especially specialists, tend to focus on only one of these in each patient. Thus it is relatively common for patients attending a hypertension clinic not to have their plasma lipids measured or for patients attending a lipid clinic not to have hormone replacement therapy even considered as a treatment option. We believe that prevention demands an integrated approach and to emphasize this point we have coined the phrase 'a pentagon of protection'. In each chapter we have reviewed the cardioprotective evidence for each drug. We have not tried to be comprehensive but have aimed to be clinically helpful.

# Acknowledgements

A book requires the involvement of many people to bring it to successful fruition; the authors are often incidental compared with the efforts of others. We must thank Debbie Eaton for her continual and cheerful help despite the succession of rewrites and last-minute changes to the final manuscript; to Iris Rajman for her constant encouragement and help with figures; and to Beverley Hughes and Isobel Clarke for their ever accommodating assistance with illustrations. At Martin Dunitz Ltd, we owe a great debt to Alan Burgess. His constant supply of good humour kept us sane at our most insecure moments and impelled us forward during times of hesitation. Finally, during our long and sometimes animated discussions about the interpretation of clinical trial data, Dr Rosemary Kendall provided an essential reminder that, irrespective of our often staunchly held opinions, our focus should not be deflected from the reason for this enterprise: the patient at risk from coronary heart disease.

## Chapter 1
# What is a cardioprotective drug?

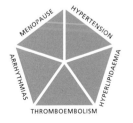

Coronary artery disease (CAD) is the most common cause of death in the developed countries of the world. It occurs more often and at an earlier age in men. Reducing the mortality and morbidity from this condition is one of the most important challenges for medicine. In some developed countries, the mortality rate is falling, partly because our knowledge about risk factors is increasing and preventive measures can be taken, and partly because medical and surgical treatment of patients with known coronary disease has improved. However, the reasons for the improvement cannot be fully explained. Some developed countries still have a high coronary mortality, and some developing countries tend to see more coronary disease, with many patients remaining unrecognized.

Up to half of all myocardial infarctions (MIs) are silent, being recognized only from the changes noted when serial electrocardiograms are performed on cohorts of patients who are under surveillance.[1] These patients are believed to have the same prognosis as those who have a clinically apparent infarction.[2] They are therefore at a considerable risk of recurrence, of sudden death, or of developing cardiac failure. Most of these patients remain undiagnosed and are therefore offered no treatment.

CAD is also an important cause of sudden death. In at least one in six instances, sudden death is the first, last and only manifestation of CAD.[3] The risk is greatest in hypertensives, smokers, those with left ventricular hypertrophy, and patients who have recovered from their first MI. Unless skilled help is immediately available, no form of treatment is possible.

The large numbers of patients with coronary disease who have silent infarctions or who die suddenly can only be reduced if at-risk patients are identified and preventive measures are undertaken. Efforts directed at the classic 'heart-attack' patient admitted to hospital can only assist a small proportion with coronary disease and can therefore only have a modest impact on total mortality and morbidity. To have a substantial impact, effective prophylactic measures are needed to prevent or delay the development of occlusive coronary disease and to reduce the risk of developing ventricular fibrillation.[4] Progress will only be made if our understanding of the pathological processes involved in endothelial damage, atheroma development, thrombus formation and plaque rupture translates into more effective means of limiting their effects. Measures should include the preferential use of drugs that may favourably influence underlying pathology.

These should be directed especially at those individuals known to be at increased risk because of, for example, hypertension or hyperlipidaemia, and those known to have coronary disease because of their past history or current symptoms.

The potential to improve the prognosis of patients known to be developing or to have CAD by appropriate drug use will only be realized if drugs with cardioprotective actions are available, if doctors are aware of the relative cardioprotective potential of the drugs they use, and if physicians are positively influenced by this property of the drug when making their choice of therapy. In practice, many doctors are often unaware of the cardioprotective potential of the drugs they use and they undervalue this property of the agents they prescribe. The aim of this book is to overcome this obstacle to effective cardioprotective therapy.

# ■ THE ISCHAEMIC CYCLE

The complexity of the processes that lead to a narrowing of the coronary arteries, and ultimately to the death of a patient, makes a detailed and comprehensive analysis of the possible sites for drug action impossible. However, one can describe in simple broad terms the important changes that can take place. These are shown in Figure 1.1, modified from Dzau and Braunwald,[5] and will form a basis for considering the effects of the drugs that we shall discuss.

Risk factors for CAD combine to influence progression towards atherosclerosis and left ventricular hypertrophy. A range of ischaemic myocardial syndromes then ensues, which ultimately lead to an MI if no intervention takes place. Through several processes – neurohumoural activation, reperfusion injury and ischaemic necrosis – remodelling produces ventricular dilatation and further left ventricular dysfunction. Heart failure progresses and either an inexorable decline continues or the patient dies suddenly. Sudden death is also an important complication in the early phase after an MI.

We will refer to Figure 1.1 at the end of each chapter as a means of indicating where existing drugs have cardioprotective actions and where further research is urgently indicated. These

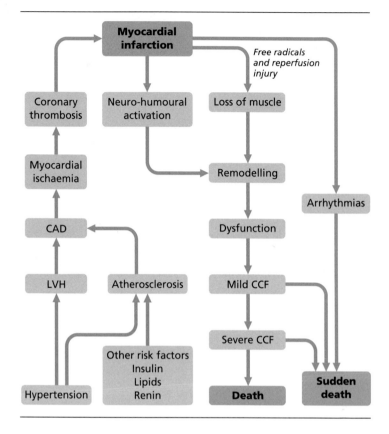

**Figure 1.1** The ischaemic cycle. CAD, coronary artery disease; LVH, left ventricular hypertrophy; CCF, chronic cardiac failure.

effects will be brought together in the final chapter, where an overall – and, we believe, optimistic – picture of cardioprotection will be presented.

## ☐ Cardioprotection

The use of the term 'cardioprotective drug' has fallen into disrepute, since it sounds like a marketing term that could be used without clearly defining its meaning and without providing

- **Impact on mechanisms**
  Does the drug reduce
  (a) Endothelial damage?
  (b) Atheroma formation?
  (c) Plaque rupture?
  (d) Thrombus formation?
  (e) The risk of developing ventricular fibrillation?

- **Clinical data**
  Does the drug reduce the risk of myocardial infarction or death:
  (a) Before the first infarction? Primary prevention.
      At–risk patient groups e.g. patients with
        Hypertension
        Angina
        Hyperlipidaemia
  (b) At the time of their infarction?
  (c) After their infarction? Secondary prevention.
      In the short term
      In the long term

Evidence that a drug is cardioprotective.

evidence to support its use. We have used the term to denote a drug that reduces the morbidity and mortality from CAD. A patient on a cardioprotective agent should be less likely to have an MI, to reinfarct, or to die suddenly from underlying coronary disease. Drugs that reduce coronary mortality by reducing deaths from heart failure in patients with ischaemic heart disease will also be discussed, but the term cardioprotective drug will be limited to the definition given above.

To make a case that a drug is cardioprotective requires evidence, first that it has actions that would enable it to modify the processes leading to death from CAD, and second that there are adequate trial data to show that the drug has an impact on coronary mortality and morbidity in clinical practice.

The Ischaemic Cycle **5**

Laboratory animal models have shown that stress, hypertension, free radicals and other pathological processes will lead to endothelial damage that may be a precursor for atheroma formation. Animals on atherogenic diets have been used to study atheroma formation, plaque rupture and thrombosis. A cardioprotective drug would be expected to have some positive beneficial effect on one or more of these pathological processes.

From a patient-oriented perspective the interpretation of clinical trial data has developed into a major component of epidemiology and an extremely important contributor to advances in therapeutics. This subject also provokes a great deal of controversy over statistical methods, data analysis, the selection of trials to be published, and bias in the inclusion of trials for meta-analysis. Although we do not propose to enter this minefield, we will draw some practical conclusions that may assist readers.

In the Western world, pathological studies and clinical evidence suggest that CAD begins in early adult life or even earlier. Those who smoke, have positive family histories, a high blood pressure or hyperlipidaemia have more severe atheroma that involves an increasing proportion of the coronary circulation, and which gradually narrows one or more vessels. When a critical narrowing develops, the patient has an MI. If they recover, the disease progresses until an occlusion at another site occurs and the patient reinfarcts or dies. This pattern of events suggests that CAD is a continuous process, and it is reasonable to believe that any intervention which prevents the second infarction ought really to reduce the risk of having a first.

The second important observation is that because coronary disease is multifactorial and takes many years to develop, the modification of one contributing factor for a short time may not have an easily demonstrable impact. This would be especially true if the abnormality in question was mild and the patient population was at low risk. Thus, to demonstrate a therapeutic effect by reducing the blood pressure of mildly hypertensive, middle-aged females would be extremely difficult, and would require such large numbers of patients as to be practically impossible in a single clinical trial.

The third difficulty is that, as indicated above, many first infarctions present as sudden death or as a silent infarction. Unless all the patient population are accounted for and unless all have an ECG at the beginning and the end, the database could be very inadequate.

Secondary prevention trials are easier to perform, since a well-defined at-risk population with a relatively high mortality and morbidity is being studied. At the very least, data from these trials strongly support the case for or against a primary prevention role for a particular form of treatment. Failure to show this in primary prevention trials may be because the trial was too small, the treatment period was too short, the patient population was at low risk, or the follow-up data were incomplete.

## ■ THE PENTAGON OF PROTECTION

We have not written this book with the intention of producing a random collection of pharmacological facts that should be applied on an ad hoc basis to the patient with ischaemic heart disease.

We see cardioprotective therapeutics as the integrated pharmacological approach to long-term management of the patient with CAD. Thus, we have introduced the notion of a pentagon of protection around the heart. That is, we have identified five aspects of therapeutic management that the clinician must consider in every patient (Figure 1.2). These are:

- hypertension
- hyperlipidaemia
- thromboembolism
- arrhythmias
- menopause

Methods of preventing, ameliorating or treating the effects of these processes may be seen to form a protective ring – the pentagon of protection – around the at-risk heart. Each patient should be given an individually tailored management strategy based on this concept – i.e. each side of the pentagon should be investigated and assessed to determine its contribution to the overall ischaemic risk and a strategy for intervention must be planned for each factor. The pentagon reinforces the idea that these important influences are not mutually exclusive; they are interdependent, with intervention in one area likely to affect the

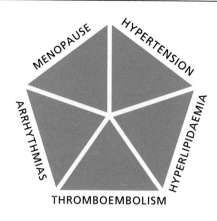

**Figure 1.2** The pentagon of protection.

imperative for intervening in another; for example, hormone replacement therapy may ameliorate a lipid profile to such a degree that specific lipid-lowering treatment is not required. The pentagon can be easily incorporated into the follow-up notes of patients with CAD and serves as a reminder of the goals of treatment.

## References

**1.** Wikstrand J, Warnold I, Toumilehto J et al, Metoprolol versus thiazide diuretics in hypertension. Morbidity results from the MAPHY study, *Hypertension* (1991) **17**:579–88.

**2.** Kannel WB, Abbott RD, Incidence and prognosis of unrecognised infarction: an update on the Framingham study, *N Engl J Med* (1984) **311**:1144–47.

**3.** Kannel WB, Cupples LA, D'Agostino RB et al, Hypertension antihypertensive treatment and sudden coronary death: the Framingham study, *Hypertension* (1988) **II**(Suppl II):45–50.

**4.** Skinner JE, Regulation of cardiac vulnerability by the cerebral defence system, *J Am Coll Cardiol* (1985) **5**:88B–94B.

**5.** Dzau V, Braunwald E, Resolved and unresolved issues in the prevention and treatment of coronary artery disease: a workshop consensus statement, *Am Heart J* (1991) **121**:1244–63.

# Chapter 2
# Hypertension

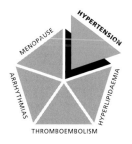

# ■ BETA-ADRENOCEPTOR BLOCKING DRUGS (BETA-BLOCKERS)

Beta-blockers probably come closest to meeting the criteria for being accepted as cardioprotective drugs. However, the available evidence is confusing because not all beta-blockers are equally effective and because, with the benefit of hindsight, primary prevention trials were not well designed. Nevertheless a case can be made that beta-blockers, and perhaps especially lipophilic beta-blockers, are cardioprotective; they have an impact on the pathological processes leading to death from coronary disease, and there are clinical trial data that (1) suggest a role in primary prevention, (2) show an impact at the time of infarction, and (3) provide clear evidence of secondary prevention.

## ☐ Mechanisms

### Endothelial injury

Haemodynamic factors cause endothelial damage and determine the sites of injury and subsequent atheroma formation. High blood pressure,[1,2] tachycardia[3] and a stressed personality[4] predispose to coronary disease, and atheromatous lesions tend to form at sites of wall stress and high turbulence.[5,6] Beta-blockers lower blood pressure, reduce heart rate, reduce the peripheral responses to stress and counteract the tendency for lesions to form at branching sites in arteries.[7]

Although several investigators have used different models to study the impact of beta-blockers on endothelial damage, the experiments of Kaplan and colleagues on stressed monkeys are most relevant. Dominant monkeys become stressed if they are required to keep establishing their dominance over other monkeys when moved from group to group. Such animals develop endothelial damage which may be prevented by either propranolol[8] or metoprolol.[9] Spence and colleagues[10] provided further evidence by assessing the effects of hypertension and high-cholesterol diet on rabbits. Propranolol was much more effective than hydralazine in reducing the aortic surface area affected by atheroma.

### Atheroma formation

There is some evidence to suggest that most antihypertensive drugs can reduce atheroma formation. The data on beta-blockers are more extensive and more impressive.[11,12] Kaplan and colleagues[11] reviewed 13 studies, in 11 of which beta-blockers (mostly propranolol) reduced atheroma formation in animals. The impact of beta-blockers was not related to blood pressure reduction and occurred despite small adverse effects on plasma lipids. It is not yet clear how beta-blockers achieve their effects but it is probably partly by reducing lipid binding to damaged endothelium,[7] perhaps by modifying the binding to arterial wall proteoglycans.[13]

### Plaque rupture
There are no data to support the belief that the risk of plaque rupture may be reduced by decreasing the haemodynamic strains imposed by high blood pressure and rapid heart rates. Nevertheless, it seems a reasonable hypothesis that beta-blockers may reduce the risk.[14]

### Thrombus formation
Beta-blockers may reduce platelet aggregation,[15,16] increase prostacyclin formation[17] and favourably modify the fibrinolytic system.[18]

### Infarction size
The consensus view is that beta-blockers reduce infarction size. Studies that have failed to show this effect have often been performed on unsuitable laboratory animal models or beta-blockers were given too late. There is a substantial quantity of animal data,[19] but the most impressive information comes from large-scale human studies.[20–23]

### Ventricular fibrillation
Ventricular fibrillation (VF) tends to occur when myocardial ischaemia is associated with high sympathetic drive and low vagal tone.[24] Beta-blockers do have anti-ischaemic effects as set out above and do protect from the effects of sympathetic drive. Until recently the possibility that lipophilic beta-blockers may have an effect on vagal tone by an action on autonomic centres in the brain was not appreciated. There are now data to show that low doses of propranolol given into the cerebral ventricles reduce the risk of VF in a stressed-pig model.[25] It has also been shown that in the dog with left ventricular hypertrophy, blood pressure reduction with metoprolol but not with enalapril reduces the risk

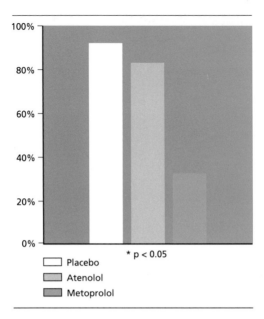

**Figure 2.1**
The incidence of ventricular fibrillation (%) in rabbits.[27]

of VF in response to acute coronary occlusion.[26] Finally, in a rabbit model rendered vulnerable by chloralose anaesthesia and acute coronary occlusion, metoprolol but not atenolol reduced the risk of VF[27] (Figure 2.1). The effect of metoprolol was shown to be related to its capacity to increase vagal tone.[27] These three animal models demonstrating the effects of beta-blockers are of considerable interest, though their relevance to human beings is open to question. Nevertheless, they help to explain the impact on sudden death in one primary prevention trial,[28] in three secondary prevention trials[21,29,30] and in two clinical studies on the incidence of VF.[31,32]

## □ Clinical data

### Primary prevention
There have been three major primary prevention trials in middle-aged hypertensives and five trials in the elderly (Table 2.1). The

**Table 2.1** Primary prevention trials.

| Patient type | Name | Year of publication | Drugs used | Impact on coronary mortality |
|---|---|---|---|---|
| **Middle-aged** | MRC[33] | 1988 | Thiazide<br>Propranolol | None |
| | IPPPSH[35] | 1985 | Oxprenolol | Reduced in non-smoking males |
| | HAPPHY[36] | 1985 | Atenolol/metoprolol<br>Thiazide | None |
| | MAPHY[37,38] | 1987 | Metoprolol<br>Thiazide | Decreased |
| **Elderly** | EWPHE | | Thiazide/triamterene<br>Thiazide | None |
| | Coope and Warrender[45] | 1991 | Atenolol/diuretic<br>Placebo | None |
| | SHEP[46] | 1991 | Chlorthalidone | None |
| | STOP[47] | 1992 | Beta-blocker/thiazide<br>Placebo | Reduced |
| | MRC[40] Elderly | 1992 | Atenolol<br>Placebo<br>Thiazide | None<br>Reduced |

trials in which beta-blocker therapy was used will be mentioned briefly, concentrating on the information they provide about the capacity of beta-blockers to prevent major coronary events. Data on total mortality are presented in Figure 2.2. Coronary events and sudden deaths are presented in Figure 2.3.

### MRC (1985) Trial[33]

The aim of this trial was to compare the effects of propranolol, a thiazide diuretic, and placebo on middle-aged hypertensives of either sex; 17 354 patients were entered into the study. The overall rates for coronary events per 1000 patient years were: propranolol 4.8, bendrofluazide 5.6, and placebo 5.5. These results were not significantly different from each other; in relation to coronary disease this trial was judged to have had a negative result. It did not produce evidence to support the belief that a beta-blocker would reduce the coronary event rate.

Unfortunately the MRC trial had three main defects. First, since there was a placebo group the patient population had mild hypertension (diastolic blood pressure 90–109 mmHg). It would have been unethical to deny active treatment to anyone with more severe hypertension. However, 18 per cent of placebo patients were normotensive on their first three annual visits and many more were intermittently normotensive. It is difficult to demonstrate a coronary preventive effect by modifying one risk factor that was only present in a proportion of patients. Second, about half the population was female. In this group the risk of a coronary event was about 1.7 per 1000 patient years, and this risk was halved in non-smokers. It is difficult to imagine reducing the risk of a coronary event from about 0.8 per 1000 patient years. Finally, a minority of major coronary events are easily recognized. To assess the impact of treatment, good data on overt coronary events, silent infarctions, and all sudden cardiac deaths are needed. In a post hoc analysis, with all the potential for bias that this entails, propranolol did reduce the risk of cardio-vascular events in non-smokers and, when silent infarctions were included, propranolol did significantly reduce the coronary event rate.[34]

### The IPPPSH trial[35]

The International Prospective Primary Prevention Study in Hypertension aimed to compare an antihypertensive regimen based on the beta-blocker oxprenolol with one not containing a

**a) Propranolol, oxprenolol and metoprolol**

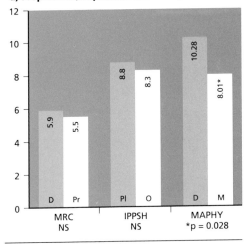

**b) Atenolol studies**

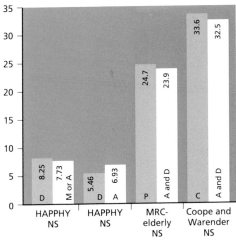

D = Diuretics, M = Metoprolol, A = Atenolol
P = Placebo, C = Control, Pr = Propranolol, O = Oxprenolol

**Figure 2.2**   Total mortality rates per 1000 patient years: (a) propranolol, oxprenolol and metoprolol; (b) atenolol studies. D = diuretics; M = metoprolol; A = atenolol; P = placebo; C = control; Pr = propranolol; O = oxprenolol.

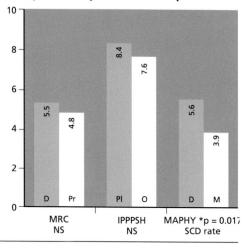

a) Propranolol, oxprenolol and metoprolol

- D = diuretics (MRC: 5.5)
- Pr = propranolol (MRC: 4.8)
- Pl = placebo (IPPPSH: 8.4)
- O = oxprenolol (IPPPSH: 7.6)
- D = diuretics (MAPHY: 5.6)
- M = metoprolol (MAPHY: 3.9)

MRC — NS
IPPPSH — NS
MAPHY *p = 0.017 SCD rate

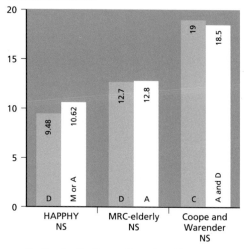

b) Atenolol studies

- D = diuretics (HAPPHY: 9.48)
- M or A (HAPPHY: 10.62)
- D = diuretics (MRC-elderly: 12.7)
- A = atenolol (MRC-elderly: 12.8)
- C = control (Coope and Warender: 19)
- A and D (Coope and Warender: 18.5)

HAPPHY — NS
MRC-elderly — NS
Coope and Warender — NS

D = Diuretics, M = Metoprolol, A = Atenolol
Pl = Placebo, C = Control, Pr = Propranolol, O = Oxprenolol

**Figure 2.3** Coronary events rate (sudden cardiac death, non-fatal MI: (a) propranolol, oxprenolol and metoprolol; (b) atenolol studies. D = diuretics; Pr = propranolol; O = oxprenolol; M = metoprolol; A = atenolol; C = control; Pl = placebo.

beta-blocker in a population of mild-to-moderately hypertensive men and women. This trial failed to yield a clear-cut result but, as in the MRC trial, the beta-blocker regimen was associated with fewer cardiac events in men. In male non-smokers the impact on critical cardiac events (5.4 versus 11.6 per 1000 patient years) in favour of oxprenolol was impressive. However, dredging data in this way may be misleading and it is noteworthy that females seemed to fare less well on oxprenolol.

### The HAPPHY–MAPHY trial[36]

This trial has been a major source of controversy and its findings have not been accepted by many. However, the results of later studies and other investigations lend some support to its original conclusions.

The trial was originally devised in 1977 as a comparison between metoprolol and a thiazide in males with moderate hypertension. By 1979 atenolol had become available and therefore other centres were recruited in which atenolol was compared with a thiazide in the belief that the two cardioselective beta-blockers would behave similarly. In 1985, at a time when some of the atenolol centre patients had only been in the trial a short time, it was decided to analyse the results, combining the atenolol and metoprolol data and comparing them with the thiazide results from all centres. Overall, beta-blockers did not reduce either total mortality (Figure 2.2) or coronary events (Figure 2.3) when compared with thiazides.[36] It therefore seemed to be a negative trial and thus, taken in conjunction with the overall results of the MRC and IPPPSH trials, strongly suggested that beta-blockers were not cardioprotective.

Following the initial analysis and without knowing the results for the individual beta-blockers, a controversial decision was made that the metoprolol/thiazide centres would continue to recruit and to monitor the progress of their patients. These data were subsequently published as the MAPHY trial and showed that metoprolol reduced overall mortality, coronary mortality,[37] sudden deaths[28] and coronary morbidity.[38]

Many found it inexplicable and therefore unacceptable that metoprolol should seem to be cardioprotective though atenolol was not. In addition, most regarded the notion of continuing to monitor one subgroup after an initial analysis had been performed as not abiding by the rules of clinical trial methodology. Nevertheless, subsequent data have not shown that atenolol is cardioprotective.[39,40] Fierce arguments against[41,42] and in favour[43,44] of the MAPHY trial have been presented.

### *Drug trials in the elderly*

Trials of primary prevention in the elderly contribute little to this subject and merit brief mention, with the exception of EWPHE, which did not involve beta-blockers. Coope and Warrender[45] showed that it was worth treating elderly hypertensives with atenolol alone or with a diuretic to reduce the risk of stroke but there was little impact on coronary mortality. The SHEP trial[46] evaluated the role of a thiazide diuretic to which atenolol could be added in patients with isolated systolic hypertension. It showed that antihypertensive therapy very effectively reduced stroke risk but also showed that most cardiovascular deaths are due to coronary disease (132/202) and many (91/202) are sudden deaths. These latter are not reduced by thiazides (with or without atenolol).

In the STOP–Hypertension trial,[47] elderly patients with hypertension were given either a beta-blocker (80 per cent) or a diuretic. Beta-blockers included metoprolol, atenolol and pindolol. Treatment reduced total mortality but also seemed to reduce coronary mortality and sudden death. However, in the MRC elderly trial,[40] although active treatment reduced the risk of stroke, atenolol again failed to have an impact on coronary disease.

In conclusion, although the primary prevention data on beta-blockers are unsatisfactory for several reasons, in the groups that are especially vulnerable – namely, middle-aged hypertensive men – a lipophilic beta-blocker may have beneficial effects on coronary mortality[33–35,37] (Figures 2.2(a) and 2.3(a)) when compared with atenolol[39,40,45] (Figures 2.2(b) and 2.3(b)). In the elderly, coronary mortality remains a serious risk,[45,46] and thiazides with or without atenolol may[40,46] or may not[45] reduce myocardial infarction rates but do not reduce the risk of sudden death.[46]

## Secondary prevention

Beta-blockers have been given both acutely and long term. In the former case the drug is usually given intravenously within a few hours of onset of symptoms suggestive of MI. Treatment may be continued for a few days or a few weeks. Long-term therapy is given orally and continued for months or even years.

### Acute studies

Many small studies and two large trials have been performed.[48] In ISIS-1,[49] 16 105 patients were randomized to receive atenolol or placebo. Atenolol reduced mortality significantly by about 14 per cent, the impact being mainly during the initial 24–48 h post infarction and due in large measure to a reduction in cardiac rupture. In the other large study, the MIAMI trial,[50] 5778 patients were randomized to either metoprolol or placebo. The overall reduction in mortality was comparable (–13 per cent) but this was not statistically significant; the effect was not limited to the initial 1–2 days and was most marked in the patients at greater risk.[46] The results of these trials are summarized in Figure 2.4.

### Chronic studies

Over 50 000 individuals have been entered into trials designed to assess the effects of chronic beta-blockade in postinfarction patients. The benefits of beta-blockers are well known, although their use is not as widespread as might be expected.

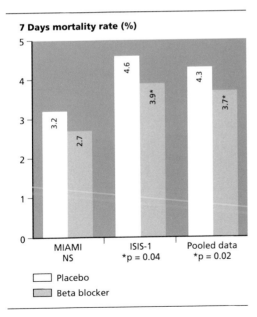

**7 Days mortality rate (%)**

**Figure 2.4**
Acute post-infarction beta-blocker studies.

MIAMI NS — 3.2 (Placebo), 2.7 (Beta blocker)
ISIS-1 *p = 0.04 — 4.6 (Placebo), 3.9* (Beta blocker)
Pooled data *p = 0.02 — 4.3 (Placebo), 3.7* (Beta blocker)

☐ Placebo
▨ Beta blocker

The Norwegian timolol study[29] was a landmark clinical trial; 4155 patients from a catchment population equivalent to one-third of Norway were enrolled 6–27 days postinfarction. The study was double blind and the patients were followed for a mean 17 months.

One hundred and eighty-four patients died whilst either on treatment or within 28 days of withdrawal. Ninety-three per cent of deaths were cardiac and 77 per cent were sudden. Timolol reduced total mortality (Figure 2.5) and cardiac mortality, dramatically reduced the rates for sudden death by 44.6 per cent ($P = 0.0001$) (Figure 2.6), and also reduced reinfarction rates. The positive effects on sudden death were maintained throughout the study and infarction rates were reduced over at least the first 6 months. Furthermore, not only did older patients, i.e. those aged 65–75 years, tolerate the treatment, but also those on active therapy had a lower mortality ($n = 28$ versus $n = 9$) and a lower infarction rate ($n = 33$ versus $n = 69$).

The Gothenberg metoprolol trial[21] differed from the Norwegian trial in that the study lasted for 3 months, but in this case the

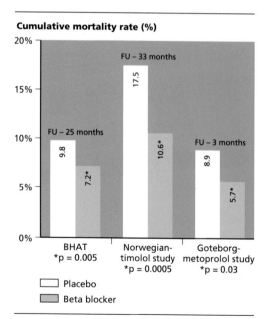

**Figure 2.5** Secondary prevention (chronic studies): cumulative mortality (%). FU = mean follow-up.

beta-blocker (metoprolol) was given intravenously as soon as possible after admission. The number of patients entering the study was 1395, and 40 (5.7 per cent) on metoprolol and 62 (8.9 per cent) on placebo died – a significant difference. Beta-blocker therapy reduced total mortality (Figure 2.5) and had a striking impact on sudden death, with a substantial reduction in episodes of VF. Metoprolol was well tolerated. The beneficial effect on sudden death has been confirmed in other studies[51] (Figure 2.6).

The Beta-blocker Heart Attack Trial (BHAT)[30] was a large US study in which 3837 patients were given propranolol or placebo, starting on average 13 days postinfarction with a mean follow-up of 25 months. Again, mortality (7.2 versus 9.8 per cent) (Figure 2.5) and sudden death (3.3 versus 4.6 per cent) (Figure 2.6) were significantly diminished.

These three studies, together with many others (see review by Yusuf and colleagues[52]), provide unequivocal evidence for the cardioprotective role of beta-blockers (Figure 2.7). Interestingly, but controversially, evidence suggests that there might be an efficacy advantage with lipophilic beta-blockers.

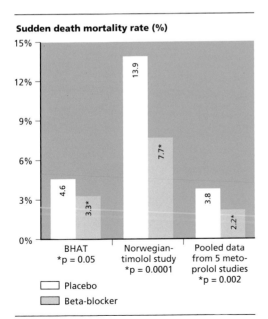

**Sudden death mortality rate (%)**

BHAT
*p = 0.05

Norwegian-timolol study
*p = 0.0001

Pooled data from 5 metoprolol studies
*p = 0.002

Placebo
Beta-blocker

**Figure 2.6**
Secondary prevention (chronic studies): sudden cardiac death mortality rate (%).

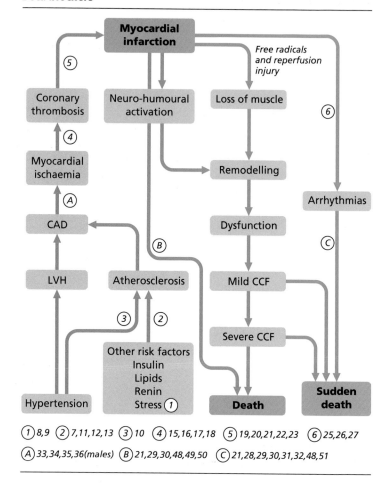

**Figure 2.7** Sites of action of beta-blockers. Animal data (numbers), clinical data (letters), relevant references as follows: (1) 8, 9; (2) 7, 11, 12, 13; (3) 10; (4) 15, 16, 17, 18; (5) 19, 20, 21, 22, 23; (6) 25, 26, 27; (A) 33, 34, 35, 36 (males); (B) 21, 29, 30, 48, 49, 50; (C) 21, 28, 29, 30, 31, 32, 48, 51.

# ■ ACE INHIBITORS

ACE inhibitors are widely used to treat hypertension and heart failure, and are likely to be increasingly prescribed to post-infarction patients. Their capacity to reduce angiotensin II (A2) concentrations and thereby allow vasodilatation and reduce fluid retention is well accepted. However, they have not been considered to be cardioprotective in the sense of having the ability to reduce the incidence, severity and consequences of coronary occlusive events. This has been despite potentially cardioprotective actions that have been thought of considerable interest but of doubtful clinical relevance. Recent data from the SAVE study,[53] which have demonstrated a capacity to reduce reinfarction rates in postinfarction patients have confirmed evidence for lower infarction rates in the SOLVD study,[54,55] in V-HeFT-II[56] and in the HY-C trial.[57] ACE inhibitors reduced the risk of sudden death. Data on mechanisms need to be reviewed and the clinical data supporting the notion that ACE inhibitors are cardioprotective drugs now merit careful scrutiny.

## ☐ Mechanisms of action

ACE inhibitors may modify the processes that lead to death from coronary artery disease (CAD) at several different sites[58] (Figure 2.8). These include:

- Impact on the renin–angiotensin system (RAS)
- Improvement in insulin sensitivity
- Inhibition of some early processes in atheroma formation
- Regression of left ventricular hypertrophy and remodelling of the myocardium
- Reduction in tissue A2-induced vasoconstriction
- Scavenging free radicals
- Reducing the incidence of arrhythmias

### Impact on the renin–angiotensin system
Increased plasma renin activity is an independent marker for increased risk of MI in patients with hypertension.[59] In a prospective study involving 1717 patients with moderate hypertension, the risk of MI was greatest in patients with high renin–sodium profiles. Despite comparable reduction in blood pressure in all

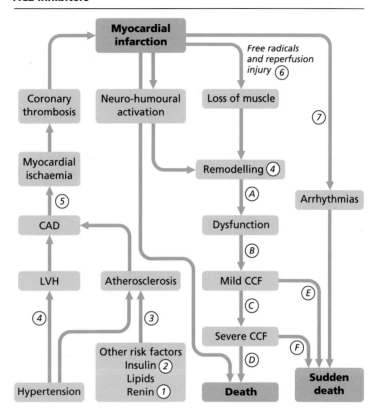

Sites of action – animal data (numbers), clinical data (letters) with the relevant references indicated below

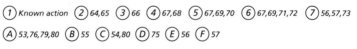

①Known action ②64,65 ③66 ④67,68 ⑤67,69,70 ⑥67,69,71,72 ⑦56,57,73
Ⓐ53,76,79,80 Ⓑ55 Ⓒ54,80 Ⓓ75 Ⓔ56 Ⓕ57

**Figure 2.8** Sites of action of ACE inhibitors. Animal data (numbers), clinical data (letters), relevant references as follows: (1) known action; (2) 64, 65; (3) 66; (4) 67, 68; (5) 67, 69, 70; (6) 67, 69, 71, 72; (7) 56, 57, 73; (A) 53, 76, 79, 80; (B) 55; (C) 54, 80; (D) 75; (E) 56; (F) 57.

three groups, the rates of MI were 13, 5.3 and 3.3 per 1000 person-years in those with high, normal and low renin–sodium profiles, respectively. The renin profile had greatest discriminative values among men, caucasians and those at low risk (non-smoking, without hyperlipidaemia or hyperglycaemia). This finding confirms results from previous studies.[60] ACE inhibitors, a class of drugs that reduces plasma A2 and counteracts the effect of high renin concentrations, could be more protective than other hypotensive drugs.

## Insulin sensitivity

The concept that hypertension, obesity and non-insulin-dependent diabetes mellitus are interrelated disorders associated with insulin resistance,[61,62] which all predispose to CAD, perhaps because of the high insulin concentrations, is well known. However, though it is possible to link high insulin and coronary disease,[63] hyperinsulinaemia is not always atherogenic and the relevance and importance of insulin resistance is not universally accepted.

Since insulin resistance seems to predispose to atheroma formation, it seems logical to avoid exacerbating this state and, if possible, to correct it in patients with other risk factors, such as hypertension. Diuretics tend to increase insulin resistance whereas ACE inhibitors reduce it.[64,65] This might explain why diuretics do not seem to reduce the risk of coronary events, while ACE inhibitors do.

## Anti-atherosclerotic effects

A2 may participate in the control of smooth muscle cell growth and proliferation, both of which are well-known events in atherogenesis. Recent studies have shown an effect of ACE inhibitors on the development of atherosclerosis in laboratory animal models and it is possible that ACE inhibitors reduce vascular proliferation and thereby suppress the development of atherosclerosis. The clinical importance of these findings is unknown, but captopril reduced aortic cholesterol content and the percentage of aortic intimal surface covered by lesions in experimental rabbits and monkeys.[66]

## Effects on remodelling

A2 increases afterload and is believed to play a part in the development of left ventricular hypertrophy, a dangerous development that may be inhibited by ACE inhibitors.[67] Furthermore, during and after MI, A2 concentrations rise and are believed to be instrumental in the remodelling process (progressive left ventricular dilatation).[67] Although early ventricular enlargement tends to restore normal systemic haemodynamic function, further increases in ventricular cavity size have a detrimental effect on ventricular performance and survival. It is therefore important to reduce cardiac enlargement by reducing the extent of the infarction and by reducing the work of the heart. ACE inhibitors, by reducing circulating concentrations of A2, decrease the tension within the wall of the left ventricle through reduction of afterload, preload or both, and thus attenuate ventricular enlargement.[53,68]

### Reduction in tissue A2-mediated vasoconstriction

Recent evidence suggests that a tissue RAS may also exist and the existence of cardiac RAS has also been shown.[69] ACE inhibitors may block cardiac A2 production and thereby prevent coronary vasoconstriction.[15] In animals and humans, ACE inhibitors have no major effects on coronary blood flow, but in myocardial ischaemia A2 concentrations rise, and so ACE inhibitors might have a greater impact during ischaemia and increase coronary blood flow.[67,70]

Vasodilatory effects of ACE inhibitors may also be due to indirect effects, e.g. stimulation of prostaglandin synthesis[67] or potentiation of the coronary dilating effect of the neuropeptide neurotensin (probably also mediated by prostaglandins).[70]

### Free radicals

The role of free radicals in the aetiology of disease and the potential use of drugs with free-radical-scavenging activity are subjects that are complex and contentious. Most data are based on animal or in vitro studies, and clinically relevant observations are limited. However, evidence is accumulating rapidly to suggest that free radicals are an important cause of disease and that therapeutic intervention directed at reducing or controlling their activity will become an important part of patient care. Most studies on ACE inhibitors have involved captopril, and interest has centred on the possible importance of its sulphydryl group.[71,72]

Patients who develop an acute coronary occlusion undergo less myocardial damage if the period of occlusion is short and coronary flow is restored either spontaneously or as a result of thrombolysis or angioplasty. Unfortunately, reperfusion is also a potential source of harm. Arrhythmias may be provoked (and will be considered in a later chapter) or a temporary interval of myocardial dysfunction (stunning) will ensue. In vitro, isolated-organ and whole-animal studies have produced evidence that captopril may act as a scavenger for some free radicals and may reduce tissue damage associated with reperfusion.[71,72]

### ACE inhibitors and arrhythmias

ACE inhibitors are not considered to be antiarrhythmic drugs. However, there is some evidence that they reduce arrhythmias in patients with severe heart failure.[56,57] ACE inhibitors tend to reduce A2-stimulated catecholamine production, increase plasma sodium and preserve potassium concentrations (and they may increase cardiac parasympathetic activity[73]). These effects may confer some antiarrhythmic potential.

## ☐ Primary prevention

Clinical trials have not yet produced long-term prognostic data on the effects of ACE inhibitors on coronary events in hypertensive patients.

The Captopril Prevention Project (CAPPP) is an ongoing study in which 7000 patients are to be recruited and followed up for 5 years.[74] Hypertensive patients previously treated or untreated with diastolic blood pressures higher than 100 mmHg are included. The primary end-points will be cardiovascular mortality, non-fatal MI and non-fatal stroke. Captopril will be compared with beta-blockers and diuretics.

The studies on ACE inhibitors in patients with heart failure [54–57] could be seen as primary prevention trials in that they may prevent the first typical MI, although in most cases their major impact was on progressive heart failure.[54,75] However, since many of the patients with heart failure already have established CAD as the cause of their heart failure, these studies are considered under secondary prevention.

## ☐ Secondary prevention

### Acute post-MI studies

Oldroyd et al conducted a double-blind, placebo-controlled study in 99 patients admitted to hospital within 24 h of acute MI.[76] Patients receiving thrombolytic therapy were excluded. Treatment with captopril began immediately after admission and the study continued for 2 months. Captopril started within 24 h after acute MI attenuated infarction expansion and favourably influenced early left ventricular remodelling as evaluated by echocardiography.

The Cooperative New Scandinavian Enalapril Survival Study II (CONSENSUS II)[77] was conducted in 6090 patients receiving enalapril or placebo. Treatment was initiated with an intravenous infusion of enalapril within 24 h after the onset of chest pain, followed by oral enalapril. All patients received standard therapy, including analgesic agents, nitrates, beta-blockers, calcium antagonists, thrombolytic agents, aspirin, diuretics and anticoagulants as indicated. Follow-up was between 41 and 180 days. Mortality rates on enalapril were non-significantly higher throughout the study (Figure 2.9). The most frequent cause of death was progressive heart failure. There were no significant differences in the rate of sudden cardiac death (2.8 per cent for enalapril versus 2.9 per cent for placebo) or rapid cardiac death (0.8 per cent for enalapril versus 0.7 per cent for placebo) within 24 h. Long-term mortality was higher among the patients given enalapril who had hypotension after the first dose (17 per cent) than among other patients given enalapril or placebo.

## Chronic post-MI studies

Sharpe et al[78] were first to describe prophylactic postinfarction ACE inhibition in man. The captopril group showed a significant increase in ejection fraction and at 12 months there was an 8–9 per cent difference in ejection fraction from baseline between the captopril and other groups. This study demonstrated that ventricular dilatation is an adverse prognostic factor for survival in the year after infarction. Subsequently, Pfeffer et al[79] conducted a double-blind, placebo-controlled trial in 59 patients with anterior MI and ventricular ejection factor (VEF) < 45 per cent. Though the differences were not statistically significant because patient numbers were small, the conclusion was that captopril attenuated ventricular enlargement in a higher risk group.

In a much larger study by Pfeffer and colleagues (Survival and Ventricular Enlargement Trial [SAVE]),[53] 2231 postinfarction patients with left VEF < 40 per cent were included. Treatment with captopril or placebo started between 3 and 16 days after MI. Follow-up was for $42 \pm 10$ months. The key results set out in Figure 2.10 included a reduction in overall mortality from 24.6

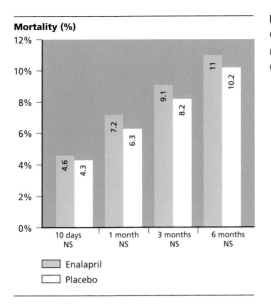

**Mortality (%)**

**Figure 2.9**
CONSENSUS II,
mortality rates
(%).

- Enalapril
- Placebo

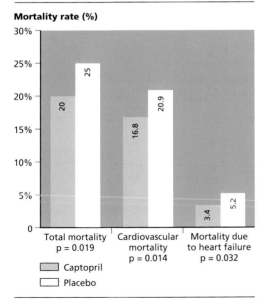

**Mortality rate (%)**

**Figure 2.10**
SAVE trial,
mortality rates (%).

- Captopril
- Placebo

ACE Inhibitors **29**

per cent to 20.4 per cent in the placebo and captopril groups, respectively. In the captopril group, 188 deaths were due to cardiovascular causes versus 234 deaths in the placebo group. This striking reduction in cardiovascular mortality was the result of the reduction in mortality due to heart failure. The reduction in the risk of progressive heart failure was 36 per cent in the captopril group. However, reinfarction (fatal or non-fatal) occurred in 170 patients in the placebo group and in 133 patients in the captopril group. Sudden cardiac death occurred in 24 patients on captopril and 25 patients on placebo.

Long-term treatment with captopril in survivors of MI with depressed left VEF but without overt heart failure resulted in reduction in total and cardiovascular mortality, the frequency of severe heart failure and recurrent MI.[53] The impact on mortality from heart failure was predictable; the reduction in reinfarction rates was surprising but did confirm the evidence from earlier studies that ACE inhibitors may have a more direct effect on coronary mortality.

The Veterans Administration Cooperative Vasodilator Heart Failure Trial II (V-HeFT-II)[56] compared the effects of enalapril with those of hydralazine and isosorbide dinitrate (ISDN) in 804 patients with chronic heart failure. Patients with active ischaemic heart disease were largely excluded, since angina limiting exercise during the bicycle ergometer test was a criterion for exclusion. Follow-up was for a mean of 2.5 years. During this interval 32.8 per cent of patients died in the enalapril group and 38.2 per cent in the hydralazine/ISDN group. Two years after the randomization, mortality in the enalapril group was significantly lower, and this trend continued throughout the study although the differences were not significant at all time points. The lower mortality in the enalapril group was due to the lower incidence of sudden cardiac death. Among enalapril recipients, 37 per cent of all deaths were from sudden cardiac events versus 46 per cent in the hydralazine/ISDN group, a difference that is statistically significant.

The so-called HY-C trial[57] was similar to V-HeFT-II in that an ACE inhibitor, in this case captopril, was compared with hydralazine. The study was performed on 117 patients with severe heart failure being assessed for cardiac transplantation. Captopril therapy significantly reduced sudden death: 3 of 44 on captopril compared with 17 of 60 on hydralazine.

The SOLVD trial (Studies of Left Ventricular Dysfunction) was conducted in two parts: first, a treatment arm[54] and second, a prevention arm.[55] The SOLVD treatment trial was conducted in 2569 patients with congestive heart failure and an ejection fraction less than 35 per cent. Approximately 90 per cent of patients were in NYHA class II and III. Follow-up was for 41.4 months. The overall mortality rate was 35.2 per cent in the enalapril group and 39.7 per cent in the placebo group (a significant risk reduction of 16 per cent). The largest reduction in cardiac deaths was among those due to progressive heart failure (risk reduction 22 per cent with enalapril). In the placebo group, the MI death rate was 4.15 per cent, and in the enalapril group it was 3.1 per cent. Enalapril, in addition to conventional therapy, significantly reduced mortality from heart failure in patients with low ejection fractions.[54] A similar study (Munich Mild Heart Failure Trial) showed that captopril also reduces the rate of deterioration in patients with NYHA class II heart failure.[80]

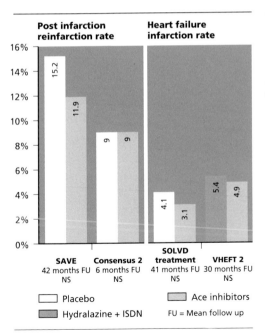

**Figure 2.11**
Infarction and reinfarction rates in four trials of ACE inhibitor therapy.

The overall cardioprotective effects of ACE inhibitors on reinfarction and infarction rates in the major trials are shown in Figure 2.11. Two trials also showed a significant reduction in sudden deaths: V-HeFT-II[4] and Hy-C.[57]

# ■ CALCIUM ANTAGONISTS

Calcium antagonists are used extensively in the management of angina and hypertension, conditions which indicate that the patient already has or is likely to develop CAD. However, though these drugs have antiatherogenic, vasodilator and antiarrhythmic properties, most clinical trials have failed to show any capacity to reduce the incidence of or mortality from CAD.

Calcium antagonists, or slow calcium channel blocking drugs, all have some effect on peripheral arteries, myocardial contractility and the cardiac conducting tissues. However, the different types of calcium antagonist differ in their impact on different tissues. Therefore it seems reasonable to consider the potential effects of the group as a whole for the various processes leading to death from CAD, whereas the clinical actions of the dihydropyridines (nifedipine-like drugs), the phenylalkylamines (e.g. verapamil) and the benzothiazepines (e.g. diltiazem) will be considered separately.

## □ Mechanisms

Calcium antagonists have been shown to have some impact on many of the processes that lead to the development of an infarction and to death from arrhythmias. Their potential to reduce atheroma formation and to encourage its regression has been a subject of particular interest.

### Atheroma Formation

Calcium deposition is a well-established part of the process leading to atheroma formation.[81,82] The more extensive the disease, the higher the calcium content, and the greater the amount of calcium, the greater the loss of the capacity to expand

and contract in response to prevailing pressures.[83] Reducing calcium deposition retards the development of atheroma.[84]

In the classic model, the cholesterol-fed rabbit, most types of calcium antagonist reduce aortic atheroma formation.[85] Nifedipine has a striking effect and isradipine is even more effective.[85] It is not clear how this benefit is achieved but possible mechanisms include reducing endothelial permeability[86] or calcium overload. These drugs may also increase cholesterol ester removal by stimulating cholesteryl ester hydrolase, modifying LDL receptors, or inhibiting matrix component synthesis and smooth muscle cell migration and proliferation.[85] All these actions are achieved independently of any antihypertensive effect of the calcium antagonist and without altering plasma lipid concentrations. Furthermore, they exert their preventive effect very early in the development of atheroma.[86,87] Calcium antagonists seem unable to delay progression of atherogenesis once it has advanced beyond the early stages.

## Thrombus formation

Calcium antagonists reduce platelet aggregation[88] but there is little evidence of any change in susceptibility to thrombus formation.

## Infarction development and size

Calcium antagonists reduce myocardial damage by partly correcting the adverse imbalance between supply and demand for oxygen and other nutrients. The different calcium antagonists to varying degrees dilate coronary arteries, modify heart rate and decrease myocardial contractility and afterload. Protection with all calcium antagonists has usually been obtained in the experimental setting when the drugs have been added before the onset of ischaemia. At a cellular level, calcium overload has been implicated as the common pathway in ischaemia-induced myocardial necrosis. Pharmacological agents that could reduce intracellular calcium concentration might protect against ischaemia and reperfusion-induced damage, but not by reducing calcium influx through slow calcium channels. Thus, the protective effects shown in experiments are probably achieved indirectly by energy sparing (negative inotropic and chronotropic effects): preservation of ATP and creatine phosphate. If sufficient ATP is available to maintain membrane ultrastructure and calcium homeostasis during ischaemia, calcium overloading will not occur on reperfusion.[89] Calcium antagonists have a protective effect on mitochondrial structure and function and they slow the release of degradative lysosomal proteases.[90]

Data from experimental coronary occlusion studies have shown that calcium antagonists reduce infarction size. The impact will depend on the nature of the coronary circulation of the animal studied, the timing of the drug dosing in relation to the coronary occlusion, the properties of the particular calcium antagonist and the methods used to determine infarction size. Dihydropyridines (particularly nifedipine), verapamil and diltiazem have all been shown to reduce infarction size.[91]

### Ventricular fibrillation

Calcium antagonists, notably verapamil and diltiazem, are effective in the management of supraventricular tachycardias, but have little or no impact on serious ventricular arrhythmias.

## ☐ Dihydropyridines

### Primary prevention

There are no convincing data to suggest that patients with either hypertension or angina are less likely to have a MI or to die if they are being treated with a dihydropyridine calcium antagonist. Some patients may even be at marginally greater risk. However, there are many studies suggesting that this group of drugs may have a positive beneficial effect on the progression of CAD.

Loaldi and colleagues[92] reported a study on angina patients treated with nifedipine, propranolol or ISDN. The progression of pre-existing lesions over a 2-year period occurred in 31 per cent on nifedipine, 53 per cent on propranolol and 47 per cent on ISDN. Furthermore, the appearance of new lesions was least on nifedipine (10 per cent) compared with propranolol (34 per cent) and ISDN (29 per cent).

The INTACT (International Nifedipine Trial on Atherosclerosis Therapy) study was designed to assess the impact of nifedipine on the progression of CAD.[93] In this relatively long-term, randomized, double-blind trial, 425 patients with mild CAD had angiographic studies before and after a 3-year course of treatment. Computer-assisted measurements showed no significant difference in the number, severity or progression of pre-existing lesions but the number of new lesions per patient was significantly fewer in those on nifedipine (28 per cent reduction). During the study active therapy did not influence the frequency of non-fatal MIs, the severity of unstable angina or the need for revascularization procedures. However, there were more cardiac deaths in those on nifedipine (8 : 2) (Figure 2.12).

The Montreal Heart Institute Study (MHIS)[94] was conducted as a double-blind placebo-controlled study in 383 patients (with 5–75 per cent stenoses in at least four coronary artery segments) treated with nicardipine or placebo. Coronary arteriography was repeated at 24 months in 335 patients. Mean progression and regression of single lesions and of disease in individual patients were not different between patients on nicardipine or placebo. But there was a significantly lower rate of progression of minor

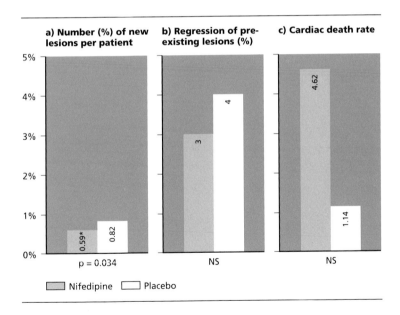

**Figure 2.12**  Results of the INTACT study: (a) number (%) of new lesions per patient; (b) regression of pre-existing lesions (%); (c) cardiac death rate.

grade stenoses (<20 per cent of luminal narrowings) in the nicardipine group compared with placebo (15 per cent versus 27 per cent of patients). Cardiac death was distributed equally between the nicardipine and placebo groups, but MI occurred more often among patients on nicardipine than placebo (14 patients with 17 MIs in the nicardipine group versus 8 patients with 9 MIs in the placebo group).

## Secondary prevention

### *Acute effects (see Figure 2.13 and Table 2.2)*
There are eight major trials assessing the impact of nifedipine given acutely after an MI.[95–102] Seven reported mortality rates are presented in Figure 2.13 and Table 2.2; the eighth[100] reported on the progression of patients with angina and threatened infarction.

The Norwegian Nifedipine Multicenter Trial[95] included 272 patients with the diagnosis of suspected MI seen within 12 h of the onset of symptoms. Definite MI developed in 67 per cent of

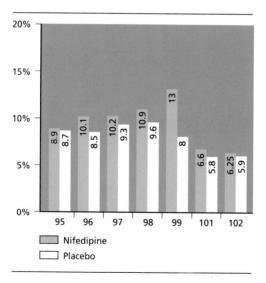

**Figure 2.13**
Mortality rate (%), acute post-MI nifedipine studies. The authors and references for each of the seven trials are presented in Table 2.2.

the nifedipine patients and in 73 per cent of the patients receiving placebo, which was not a significant difference. Infarction size was similar in both groups as well as mortality after 6 weeks.

In the Nifedipine Angina Myocardial Infarction Study,[96] 105 patients with threatened MI and 66 patients with acute MI were included and treated with nifedipine a mean of 4.6 h after the onset of symptoms. Nifedipine did not reduce the likelihood of progression from threatened MI to acute AMI, since 75 per cent of each group (nifedipine and placebo) went on to infarct. Infarction size was also similar in both groups. Two-week mortality was 7.9 per cent in the nifedipine group and 0 per cent in the placebo group. This finding raises the possibility that nifedipine exacerbated the sequelae of infarction. There was no difference in total mortality at 6 months.

The Trial of Early Nifedipine Treatment (TRENT)[97] studied 4491 patients with suspected MI. Within 24 h of the onset of symptoms, patients received treatment with oral nifedipine. In both groups 64 per cent of patients developed an acute MI during the observation period. The mortality rate in patients with confirmed MI was 10.2 per cent in the treated group versus 9.3 per cent in the placebo group. Compared with placebo, the nifedipine-treated patients were found to have significant decreases in systolic and diastolic pressure and increases in heart rate.[97]

Branagan et al[98] conducted a study that included 98 patients with suspected MI who received nifedipine or placebo approximately 3.3 h from the onset of symptoms. There were no significant differences in 1-month mortality or infarction size

| Study | Nifedipine | Placebo | Statistical significance |
|---|---|---|---|
| Sirnes et al[95] | 8.9 | 8.7 | NS |
| Muller et al[96] | 10.1 | 8.5 | NS |
| Wilcox et al[97] | 10.2 | 9.3 | NS |
| Branagan et al[98] | 10.9 | 9.6 | NS |
| Erbel et al[99] | 13.0 | 8.0 | NS |
| Walker et al[101] | 6.6 | 5.8 | NS |
| Gotlieb et al[102] | 6.25 | 5.9 | NS |

**Table 2.2**  Mortality rate (%), acute post-MI nifedipine studies.

between the two groups. Also, there was no significant difference at 1-month in the progression from the coronary insufficiency to MI.

Erbel et al[99] reported the results of a trial in 149 patients with chest pain lasting longer than 30 min, together with ECG changes, who received either nifedipine or placebo treatment immediately. All patients were given intracoronary streptokinase and, in addition, the nifedipine group were given intracoronary nifedipine before and after the thrombolytic therapy. The in-hospital mortality rate was 13 per cent in the nifedipine group and 8 per cent in the placebo group. Patients treated with nifedipine had 16 per cent incidence of reinfarction versus 11 per cent in the placebo group. Reocclusion of the infarction-related vessel occurred in 20 per cent of the nifedipine group and in 13 per cent of patients in the placebo group. None of the reported differences were significant.

Although not significant, this trend towards increased cardiovascular morbidity and mortality in nifedipine-treated patients is disturbing (Table 2.2; Figure 2.13). In other acute MI trials with nifedipine, there were no significant differences between nifedipine and placebo groups with respect to infarction size, the incidence of ventricular arrhythmias or hospital mortality.[100–102]

### Long-term effects (Table 2.3 and Figure 2.14)

The Secondary Prevention Reinfarction Israeli Nifedipine Trial (SPRINT 1)[103] included 2276 patients 7–21 days after acute MI. They were randomized to receive nifedipine or placebo over a mean duration of 10 months. The 10-month mortality rate in the placebo group was 5.75 per cent versus 5.8 per cent in the nifedipine-treated group. There was no difference in recurrent

| Study | Nifedipine | Placebo | Statistical significance |
|-------|------------|---------|--------------------------|
| SPRINT I[103] | 5.8 | 5.7 | NS |
| SPRINT II[104] | 9.3 | 9.3 | NS |

**Table 2.3**  Mortality rate (%), long-term nifedipine studies.

MI between nifedipine and placebo group (4.4 per cent versus 4.8 per cent respectively). The authors concluded that nifedipine beginning 2 or 3 weeks after the event does not reduce mortality or recurrent infarction.

In the placebo-controlled SPRINT II trial,[104] 1373 patients were randomized to receive nifedipine as soon as possible after the onset of acute MI. Follow-up was 6 months. There was no difference in mortality between the two groups (9.3 per cent in both). However, mortality was higher in nifedipine-treated patients who initially presented with low systolic blood pressure (<100 mmHg). Thus, SPRINT II extended the preliminary conclusion of SPRINT I that neither early nor late administration of nifedipine has any effect in subsequent cardiac events in survivors of MI.

Despite many theoretical reasons, some animal data and angiographic evidence of benefit, clinical studies have failed to show a benefit from calcium antagonist treatment. Long-term primary prevention studies in hypertension have not been

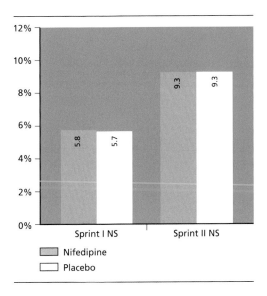

**Figure 2.14**
Mortality rate (%). Long-term nifedipine studies: SPRINT I[103] and SPRINT II.[104]

performed and short-term studies in unstable angina[105] or acutely postinfarction have been negative. Longer term postinfarction studies have not demonstrated any reduction in reinfarction or mortality. The lack of impact in the acute setting might be attributed to the vasodilatation that stimulates an increase in sympathetic nervous system activity and which is potentially counterproductive. This could be controlled by giving a dihydropyridine with a beta-blocker; there is some evidence for this notion.[100]

## ☐ Verapamil

### Primary prevention

Verapamil is a calcium antagonist with substantial antiarrhythmic properties which has been shown to have useful antiatherogenic actions in animal studies and tends to increase plasma concentrations of HDL in man.[106] However, as yet there is no good evidence that it will reduce the risk of having an MI or dying from it. There is little evidence that it has a beneficial impact on atheroma formation in man.

In the Frankfurt retrospective trial,[107] a group of 43 patients aged 40–65 years with CAD was evaluated. After the initial angiography, 26 patients received long-term therapy with verapamil and 17 patients received conventional antianginal therapy (beta-blockers and nitrates). Average follow-up was 13 months. Coronary lesions regressed in a significantly greater proportion of patients on verapamil (21 per cent) than in patients on standard therapy (8 per cent). Regression of high-grade stenosis (41 per cent) occurred significantly more frequently than regression of low-grade stenoses (12 per cent) in the verapamil group. Lower mean progression in individual stenoses and less frequent occurrence of new effective stenoses in the verapamil-treated patients were observed (3.3 per cent versus 10.9 per cent, respectively).[107]

A prospective study, the Frankfurt Isoptin Progression Study (FIPS),[86] involved 445 patients after coronary artery bypass surgery (i.e. advanced stages of CAD) who were randomized to either verapamil or placebo. Angiographic evaluations were performed 3 years after enrolment in 79 patients on verapamil and 80 patients on placebo. No significant differences were found between the two groups with regard to progression or regression of pre-existing stenoses, development of new stenoses or new occlusions in both the native vessels and bypass grafts. There were no differences in progression or regression of stenoses of low or high grade between treatment groups. Cardiac deaths (five in the verapamil group and three in the placebo group) and the need for bypass surgery were equally distributed between both groups.

The Verapamil in Hypertension Atherosclerosis Study (VHAS) is an ongoing study designed to compare verapamil slow release and chlorthalidone in lowering blood pressure, retarding atherosclerotic progression in carotid arteries in hypertensive patients and reducing cardiovascular mortality.[108] The double-blind, 3-year study includes 1464 patients with essential hypertension.

## Secondary prevention

### *Acute effects*

Crea and colleagues[109] reported the results of a single-blind placebo-controlled study in 17 patients with acute MI. They were given verapamil or placebo in an intravenous regimen. Treatment was started a mean of 6.5 h after the onset of symptoms. The study failed to prevent angina and reinfarction in patients after acute MI.

The only clinical trial reporting any benefit from verapamil given early in an acute MI was conducted by Bussman et al.[110] Fifty-four patients treated with intravenous verapamil were included. A reduction of 30 per cent in creatine kinase-MB (CK-MB) release was observed. The group on verapamil required less lignocaine and diuretic therapy than the control group. This small study was not double blind.

### *Long-term studies*

Based on the evidence of experimental studies in which verapamil has been shown to reduce infarction size, the Danish study group conducted a randomized, placebo-controlled, double-blind trial: the Danish Verapamil Infarction Trial (DAVIT-I).[111] The aim was to determine whether an intravenous bolus of verapamil followed by oral verapamil for 6 months might decrease total death and reinfarction rate. DAVIT-I included 717 patients in the verapamil group and 719 patients in the placebo group. The differences in mortality and reinfarction rates between the two groups after the 6 months were not significant.

Retrospective analysis of the data showed a lower mortality rate in the verapamil group (3.7 per cent) versus the placebo group (6.4 per cent) between days 22 and 180. The reinfarction rate was 3.9 per cent in the verapamil group compared with 7.0 per cent in the placebo group between days 15 and 180.[111] These results encouraged the authors to conduct a late intervention trial to investigate whether the treatment with verapamil from the second week after an acute MI, continued for at least 1 year, might reduce total mortality and major events (cardiac death and reinfarction).

The Danish Verapamil Infarction Trial II (DAVIT-II)[112] was also a double-blind, placebo-controlled multicentre study that included 878 patients on verapamil and 897 patients on placebo started in the second week after admission to the hospital and continued for a mean of 16 months. The 18-month cumulative mortality rate was 11.2 per cent and 13.8 per cent in the verapamil and placebo group, respectively. Sudden death rate was 5.7 per cent and 7.5 per cent and cardiac death rate was 9.9

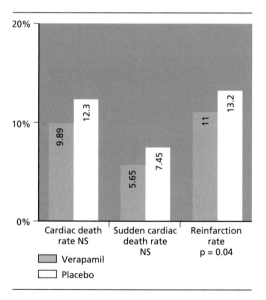

**Figure 2.15**
DAVIT-II data.[112]

per cent and 12.3 per cent in the verapamil and placebo group, respectively. These differences were not significant. However, there were 91 reinfarctions on verapamil compared with 129 in the placebo group. The 18-month first reinfarction rate was 11 per cent in the verapamil and 13.2 per cent in the placebo group. This difference was significant (Figure 2.15). In patients without heart failure, the 18-month overall mortality rate (7.7 per cent versus 11.8 per cent) and major events rate (14.6 per cent versus 19.7 per cent) were significantly reduced in the verapamil compared with the placebo group (Figure 2.16). Long-term treatment with verapamil after an MI prevents reinfarction and death with the most pronounced effects in patients without heart failure (DAVIT-II).

Verapamil has not been investigated as extensively as the beta-blockers or the dihydropyridines. Its pharmacodynamic actions and the results of DAVIT-II (and some of those DAVIT-I) suggest a long-term positive effect in secondary prevention.

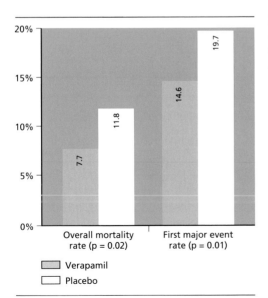

**Figure 2.16**
DAVIT-II – patients without heart failure.[112]

## ☐ Diltiazem

### Primary prevention

There are no clinical data to support the contention that dilti-azem might prevent a first infarction.

### Secondary prevention

Two trials have assessed the impact of diltiazem in MI patients and have shown benefit in the short term in those with non-Q-wave infarction and in the long-term in those with good left ventricular function. Some regard these observations as provid-ing good evidence that diltiazem has a useful cardioprotective role; others are sceptical about a drug that only seems to help a subgroup of the population at risk.

### *Acute study*

The Multicenter Diltiazem Reinfarction Study[113] included 576 patients with non-Q-wave MI (which accounts for one third of all MIs). They received diltiazem or placebo, starting 24–72 h after the onset of symptoms and continuing for 14 days. The primary end-point was reinfarction within 14 days. Secondary end-points were postinfarction angina and refractory angina. Recurrent MI was documented in 27 patients on placebo (9.3 per cent) and in 15 patients on diltiazem (5.2 per cent), which was significantly different. The 14-day mortality was similar but diltiazem reduced the frequency of refractory postinfarction angina by 49.7 per cent.

Zannad et al[114] conducted a double-blind, placebo-controlled study in 34 patients within 6 h of the onset of MI. All patients received heparin and a constant infusion of lignocaine. The dilti-azem-treated group showed a significant decrease of the infarc-tion size, although the treated group was small.

### *Long-term study*

The Multicenter Diltiazem Postinfarction Trial (MDPIT)[115] enrolled 2466 patients with MI. They received either diltiazem or placebo and were followed for 12–52 months (mean 25 months). The primary end-points were total mortality and first cardiac event (cardiac death or non-fatal MI). There were 226 cardiac events in the placebo and 202 in the diltiazem group (11 per cent reduction), which was not a statistically significant difference. There was no difference in total mortality rate. Diltiazem was associated with a significant reduction in the incidence of the cardiac events in the 1909 patients (80 per cent) who did not have pulmonary congestion. But in 490 patients (20 per cent) with pulmonary congestion, diltiazem was associated with a significant increase of cardiac events.

In patients without pulmonary congestion the cardiac event rates were 8 per cent for diltiazem and 11 per cent for placebo. In groups of patients with pulmonary congestion, cardiac event rates were 26 per cent for diltiazem and 18 per cent for placebo (Figure 2.17).

In the 68–80 per cent of patients with left VEF greater than 40 per cent, diltiazem was associated with decreased incidence of cardiac death and cardiac events rate (6 per cent versus 10 per cent). However, in patients with left VEF less than 40 per cent it was associated with a borderline statistically significant increase of cardiac death and cardiac events rate (26 per cent versus 20 per cent). Although 55 per cent of patients were also taking beta-blockers, there were no significant interactions between these treatments.[115]

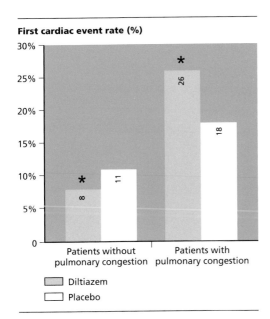

**First cardiac event rate (%)**

**Figure 2.17**
MDPIT, first cardiac event rate ($p < 0.01$).[115]

## Sites of action of calcium antagonists

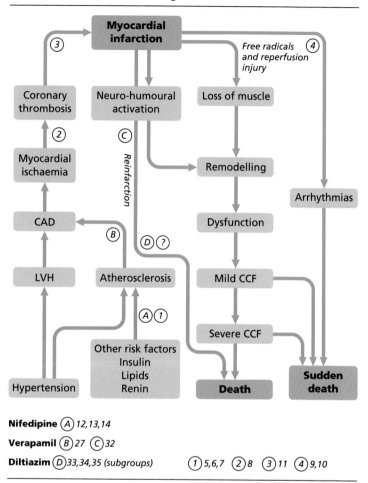

**Nifedipine** Ⓐ 12,13,14
**Verapamil** Ⓑ 27 © 32
**Diltiazim** Ⓓ 33,34,35 (subgroups)    ① 5,6,7  ② 8  ③ 11  ④ 9,10

**Figure 2.18** Sites of action of calcium antagonists. Animal data (numbers), clinical data (letters), relevant references as follows: (1) 85, 86, 87; (2) 88; (3) 91; (4) 89, 90. Nifedipine: (A) 92, 93, 94. Verapamil: (B) 107; (c) 112. Diltiazem: (D) 113, 114, 115 (subgroups).

Subgroup analysis from the MDPIT study in 634 patients with non-Q-wave infarction during a follow-up of 1-year was done. The cumulative 1-year cardiac event rate was 15 per cent in the placebo and 9 per cent in the diltiazem group. During the entire 52-month follow-up there were 67 cardiac events in the placebo group and 41 in the diltiazem group, a significant 34 per cent reduction in event rate. There was an associated 30 per cent reduction in the total mortality and cumulative 38 per cent reduction in cardiac mortality. These results show that long-term prophylactic diltiazem treatment in patients with non-Q-wave MI is associated with highly significant reduction in one-year mortality.[116]

Diltiazem seems to help some postinfarction patients; those who have a non-Q-wave infarction and those who do not develop pulmonary oedema. There are no primary prevention data. Further trials are needed to establish whether diltiazem could be considered a cardioprotective drug.

The calcium antagonists are a group of drugs which have many actions suggesting that they may have a striking impact on CAD (Figure 2.18). Clinical trial data have so far provided little evidence to suggest that these drugs are cardioprotective. There is no evidence that any of the three groups of calcium antagonists will reduce the risk of having a first coronary event, and postinfarction verapamil and diltiazem have only been shown to have an impact on patients with well-preserved cardiac function.

# ■ ALPHA-ADRENERGIC BLOCKING DRUGS

The selective postjunctional alpha$_1$-adrenergic blocking drugs (alpha-blockers), such as prazosin, doxazosin and terazosin, represent a striking improvement as antihypertensive agents compared with earlier alpha-blockers. These drugs have the potential to modify several risk factors for cardiovascular disease.

### *Effects on plasma lipid profile*
The level of cholesterol and especially the total cholesterol/HDL cholesterol ratio are considered important coronary heart disease risk factors.[117] Alpha-blockers are the only antihypertensive drugs

that produce a beneficial effect on blood lipids. Several studies have demonstrated a favourable effect of alpha₁-blocker therapy on lipid metabolism.[118–120]

Prazosin produces a fall in total triglycerides, total cholesterol, LDL cholesterol, and VLDL cholesterol and causes an increase in HDL cholesterol concentration of 2–15 per cent[121–124] (Figure 2.19). Doxazosin and terazosin have similar effects[125–127] (Figure 2.20). Doxazosin has favourable effects on lipid profiles in patients with type II diabetes mellitus and hypertension.[126,128]

A meta-analysis of the pooled data from several studies, including 5413 hypertensive patients on doxazosin, has shown significant reduction of LDL cholesterol by 4.8 per cent and triglycerides by 7.6 per cent and significant increase of the total cholesterol/HDL cholesterol ratio by 5.8 per cent[129] (Figure 2.21).

Alpha-blockers also stimulate lipoprotein lipase and lecithin:cholesterol acyltransferase (LCAT) activity,[130] which may be responsible for triglyceride reduction and HDL cholesterol increase. Leren[131] found that doxazosin stimulates LDL receptors

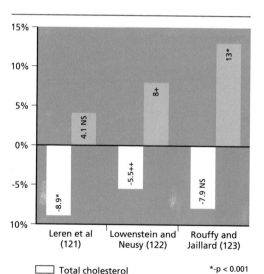

**Figure 2.19** Percentage of change from baseline of the total and HDL cholesterol with prazosin.

Total cholesterol
HDL cholesterol

*-p < 0.001
+p = 0.02
++p = 0.002

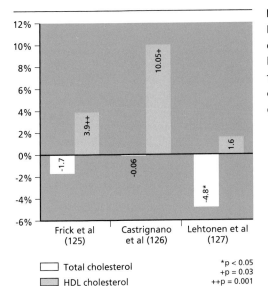

**Figure 2.20**
Percentage of change from baseline for the total and HDL cholesterol with doxazosin.

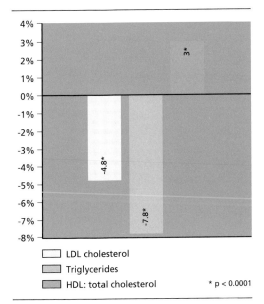

**Figure 2.21**
Pooled data on the effects of doxazosin on the LDL, triglycerides, and HDL/total cholesterol ratio.[129]
*p < 0.05.

in fibroblasts, suggesting enhanced catabolism of LDL. Alpha-blockers may also modify the adrenergic regulation of cholesterol synthesis.[132]

### *Effects on insulin sensitivity*

Insulin resistance is often associated with hypertension and type II diabetes and may lead to sodium retention and disturbances in glucose and lipid metabolism, which all increase risk for coronary heart disease.

Alpha-blockers have been shown to improve insulin sensitivity in hypertensive patients with impaired glucose tolerance and insulin resistance.[133] Prazosin significantly improved insulin-mediated glucose disposal in moderately obese hypertensive patients.[134] Furthermore, doxazosin has been shown to reduce serum levels of insulin and glucose in hypertensive patients.[127,135] These changes in blood glucose levels and serum insulin sensitivity in hypertensive patients could favourably affect the probability of developing coronary heart disease. Alpha-blockers have no impact on serum potassium or uric acid concentrations.[120]

### *Effects on ventricular hypertrophy*

Hypertension is the main cause of left ventricular hypertrophy, which has been shown to be an important independent risk factor for coronary heart disease. In hypertensive patients, treatment with prazosin,[136] doxazosin,[137] and terazosin[138] significantly reduced left ventricular mass. This reduction could be due to reduction in left ventricular wall stress as a result of decreased peripheral vascular resistance, afterload or blood pressure.

### *Antithrombotic effects of alpha-blockers*

In hypertensive patients, induced platelet aggregation is significantly reduced with doxazosin compared with placebo.[139] In 84 hypertensive patients, doxazosin improved the activity of the fibrinolytic system (tissue plasminogen activator activity significantly increased).[140]

## Primary prevention

Long-term comparative studies involving large populations have confirmed that monotherapy with prazosin, doxazosin and terazosin[122,123,137,141] produces a significant and sustained reduction in blood pressure in patients with mild-to-moderate hypertension. However, despite their beneficial effects on some risk

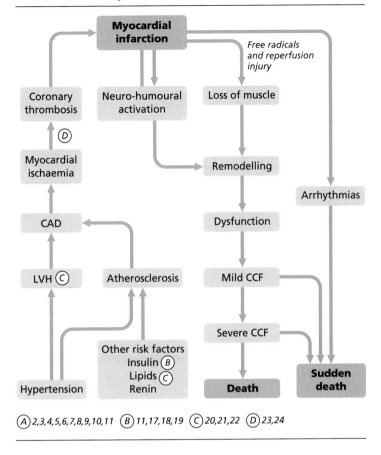

**Figure 2.22** Sites of action of alpha-blockers. Relevant references as follows: (A) 117, 118, 120, 121, 122, 123, 124, 125, 126, 127, 128; (B) 127, 133, 134, 135; (C) 136, 137, 138; (D) 139, 140.

factors there is no good evidence that alpha-blockers have produced a reduction in coronary heart disease morbidity and mortality, since the appropriate studies have not yet been done. A possible benefit of alpha-blockers in preventing coronary heart disease will only be settled after obtaining the results of long-term comparison studies of alpha-blockers with coronary heart disease morbidity and mortality as end-points (such as the TOMHS trial).[142]

There is a large database on the use of alpha-blockers in patients with heart failure. Furberg and Yusuf[143] reviewed nine trials with alpha-blockers in heart failure and concluded that they probably do not improve survival.

### Secondary prevention
Alpha-blockers are not used in postinfarction patients.

A summary of the properties of alpha-blockers is shown in Figure 2.22.

## ■ ORGANIC NITRATES

Nitrates have been used for over 100 years to relieve the pain of angina pectoris.[144] More recently, efforts have been directed to finding an effective long-acting preparation that could be used prophylactically and which is not rendered ineffective because of the development of tolerance.[145,146] In addition, intravenous nitrates are now being used extensively in the management of patients with acute MI and those with acute left ventricular failure. Not only do they relieve symptoms, but they also reduce coronary mortality.[147]

The increasing use of nitrates has been associated with and possibly, in part, caused by advances in our understanding of the many ways in which these drugs might influence CAD. The inclusion of a nitrate preparation in the ISIS-4 study[148] is evidence for the acceptance of nitrates as potentially important cardioprotective drugs.

### □ Mechanisms

The basic haemodynamic effects of nitrates are well known. However, the large number of detailed investigations performed in recent years have added greatly to our understanding of these.

Nitrates are predominantly vasodilators that reduce venous return, pulmonary oedema and heart work.[149] They also dilate peripheral arteries and lower peripheral resistance, which also reduces heart work.[150] In addition, they dilate coronary arteries, improve collateral flow, open up regions of stenotic narrowing and relax vasospasm.[151] Nitrates influence several processes that contribute to the morbidity and mortality from CAD.

## Impact on diseased vessels

Endothelium-derived relaxing factor (EDRF) acts as a vasodilator in normal vessels. The active constituent is believed to be nitric oxide or a closely related substance. When the endothelium is damaged by atheromatous disease[152] or even by hypercholesterolaemia, vasodilatation may be impaired. Organic nitrates, such as those used therapeutically, are converted in the vessel wall by various steps that include a reaction with sulphydryl groups to form nitric oxide and are thus able to act as an 'exogenous EDRF'. Furthermore, when the endothelium is damaged, nitrates seem to be more effective vasodilators[151] making them potentially valuable therapeutic agents in patients with acute or chronic myocardial ischaemia due to endothelial disease.

## Modification of platelet function

The role of nitrates as anti-aggregatory agents that tend to modify platelet function and reduce the risk of thrombus formation has been demonstrated in several studies[153-155] but remains a subject of debate.[151] Platelets play a key part in thrombus formation, often the final step in the development of a coronary occlusion. Enhanced platelet activity has been documented in patients with acute MI or unstable angina[156] and this activity tends to increase during the early hours of the day when MIs and episodes of silent ischaemia are most likely to occur.[157]

## Left ventricular remodelling

Remodelling after MI leads to wall thinning, cavity dilatation and impaired function. Left ventricular end-systolic volume is a predictor of mortality, and patients who develop large left ventricles are more prone to cardiac failure, left ventricular aneurysms and risk of death from cardiac disease. In animals and in humans, nitrates and ACE inhibitors have been shown to suppress this deleterious remodelling process.[158,159]

### Anti-ischaemic effects

Early studies at the Johns Hopkins Hospital evaluated the haemodynamic effects of intravenous nitroglycerin in patients with an acute MI.[160] Not only did the treatment improve left ventricular function but it also reduced ischaemic damage as assessed by ST-segment mapping.

Several other studies have demonstrated that infarction size may be reduced by intravenous nitroglycerin given early after the onset of symptoms of MI. Bussman and colleagues[161] compared 31 treated with 29 control patients and showed an overall 23 per cent reduction in infarction size as determined by plasma creatine kinase (CK) concentrations. Jaffe and colleagues[162] also showed a reduction in CK infarction size but only in patients with inferior infarcts. Derrida and co-workers[163] showed a beneficial impact on ECG changes, and Jugdutt and Warnica[158] again showed a decrease in CK infarction size and 3-month mortality. The effects on CK infarction size are shown in Figures 2.23 and 2.24.

The reduction in infarction size found in these studies may in part be explained by the fact that nitrates tend to improve collateral flow both in animal models[164] and in man.[165]

## ☐ Primary prevention

No data are yet available to show any primary preventive benefit of treatment.

## ☐ Secondary prevention

In 1988 Yusuf and colleagues[147] completed a meta-analysis of 10 trials of nitrate therapy (three nitroprusside, seven nitroglycerin). Most of these trials contained relatively small numbers of patients but all involved the administration of intravenous therapy started soon after the onset of symptoms associated with MI and continued for 48–72 hours. The overall result for nitroprusside was a non–significant reduction in mortality (17.8 per cent on placebo, 14.3 per cent on active therapy). Intravenous nitroglycerin produced a significant reduction in mortality (20.5 per cent on placebo, 12.0 per cent on active treatment).

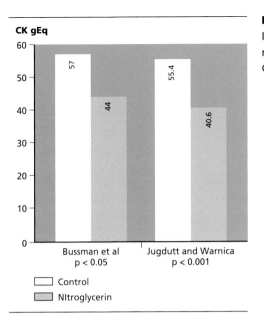

**Figure 2.23**
Impact of
nitroglycerin on
CK infarction size.

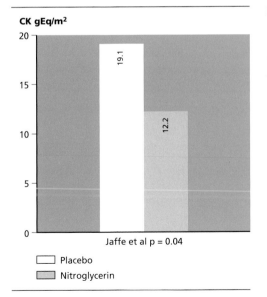

**Figure 2.24**
Impact of
nitroglycerin on
CK infarction size
after inferior
myocardial
infarction.

## Sites of action of organic nitrates

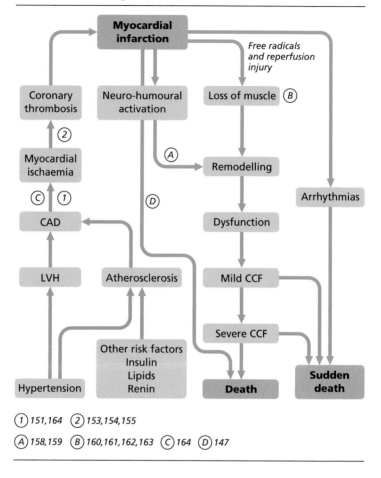

**Figure 2.25** Sites of action of organic nitrates. Animal data (numbers), clinical data (letters), relevant references as follows: (1) 151, 164; (2) 153, 154, 155; (A) 158, 159; (B) 160, 161, 162, 163; (C) 164; (D) 147.

There are no good data on the effects of longer term oral nitrate therapy but this is being addressed in the ISIS-4 trial.[148] A once-daily regimen of a controlled-release form of isosorbide 5-mononitrate was chosen because it minimizes the risk of developing tolerance.

Until recently nitrates were considered to be simple vasodilators, undoubtedly effective in the management of acute angina, but one of the least exciting groups of cardiovascular drugs. They are now seen to have several cardioprotective effects in addition to their valuable haemodynamic actions (Figure 2.25). Taken together with the results of the acute post-MI studies, it now seems that nitrates may have a more exciting future. Though it is too early to suggest that nitrates given orally long term will have a cardioprotective role in patients with angina or post-infarction, it is fairly certain that these drugs will do much more than dilate veins.

## ■ CONCLUSION

Several different classes of drugs to treat patients with hypertension and angina or those who have had an infarction have been discussed. No single preparation can claim to be the most effective, the best tolerated, the easiest to use and the most likely to prevent cardiovascular complications. Furthermore, the requirements of patients differ and the presence of other diseases and the taking of other medication will influence the choice of antihypertensive and antianginal agent. However, since major coronary events and sudden death are the most common complications of hypertension, angina and the postinfarction state, the physician should be aware of the potential of the preparations which he or she uses to reduce the patient's risk of developing these complications. All the drugs described have *some* capacity to reduce some risk factors and so should have *some* impact on the underlying disease. To date only for beta-blockers can a claim be made that they have an impact on several of the pathological processes that lead to death from CAD. In addition, there are some primary prevention data in males and convincing secondary prevention data. ACE inhibitors have several potentially beneficial effects on CAD and they seem to reduce the risk of MI in patients with heart failure and in postinfarction patients followed for long enough. Clinical data are limited for verapamil, diltiazem and nitrates and lacking for dihydropyridines and alpha-blockers.

In patients known to have hypertension or CAD, not only should appropriate treatment be offered as indicated above, but also the risks from hyperlipidaemia, thromboembolism, arrhythmias and being postmenopausal should be considered. Deaths from a multifunctional disease are unlikely to be strikingly reduced by attempting to modify one risk factor alone.

### References

**1.** Pooling Project Research Group: Relationship of blood pressure, serum cholesterol, smoking habit, relative weight and ECG abnormalities to incidence of major coronary events. Final report of the Pooling Project, *J Chron Dis* (1978) **31**:201–306.

**2.** Holme I, Enger SC, Helgeland A et al, Risk factors and raised atherosclerotic lesions in coronary and cerebral arteries. Statistical analysis from the Oslo study, *Atherosclerosis* (1981) **1**:250–6.

**3.** Kannel WB, Thomas HE: Sudden coronary death. The Framingham Study, *Ann N Y Acad Sci* (1982) Part 1: 3–20.

**4.** Disdale JE, A perspective on type A behaviour and coronary disease, *N Engl J Med* (1988) **318**:110–2.

**5.** Pettersson K, Benjne B, Bjork H, Strawn WB, Bondjers G, Experimental sympathetic activation causes endothelial injury in the rabbit thoracic aorta via B-adrenoceptor activation, *Circ Res* (1990) **67**:1027–34.

**6.** Zarins CK, Giddens DP, Bharadray BK et al, Carotid bifurcation atherosclerosis. Quantitative correlation of plaque localisation with flow velocity profiles and wall shear stress, *Circ Res* (1983) **53**:502–514.

**7.** Thubrikar MJ, Christie AM, Cao-Danh HC, Holloway PE, Nolan SP, Metoprolol reduces low density lipoprotein uptake in aortic regions prone to atherosclerosis, *FASEB J* (1990) **4**:A1151.

**8.** Kaplan JR, Manuck SB, Adams MR et al, Propranolol inhibits coronary atherosclerosis in behaviourally predisposed monkeys fed an atherogenic diet, *Circulation* (1987) **76**:1364–72.

**9.** Strawn W, Bondjers G, Kaplan JR et al, Endothelial dysfunction in response to psychosocial stress in monkeys, *Circ Res* (1991) **68**:1270–9.

**10.** Spence JD, Perkins DG, Klein RL, Adams MR, Haust MD, Hemodynamic modifications of aortic atherosclerosis: effects of propranolol versus hydralazine in hypertensive hyperlipidemic rabbits, *Atherosclerosis* (1984) **50**:325–33.

**11.** Kaplan JR, Manuck SB, Adams MR, Clarkson TB, The effects of beta-adrenergic blocking agents on atherosclerosis and its complications, *Eur Heart J* (1987) **8**:928–44.

**12.** Oslund-Lindqvist AM, Lindquist P, Brautigam J et al, The effect of metoprolol on diet-induced atherosclerosis in rabbits, *Arteriosclerosis* (1988) **8**:40–4.

**13.** Linden T, Camejo G, Wiklund O et al, Effect of short-term beta blockade on serum lipid levels and on the interaction of LDL with human arterial proteoglycans, *J Clin Pharmacol* (1990) **30**:S123–31.

**14.** Fitzgerald JD, By what means might beta-blockers prolong life after acute myocardial infarction? *Eur Heart J* (1987) **8**:945–51.

**15.** Frishman WH, Christodouou J, Weksler B et al, Abrupt propranolol withdrawal in angina pectoris: effects on platelet aggregation and exercise tolerance, *Am Heart J* (1978) **95**:169–79.

**16.** Willich SN, Pohjola-Sintonen S, Bhatia SHS et al, Suppression of silent ischaemia by metoprolol without alteration of morning increase of platelet aggregability in patients with stable coronary artery disease, *Circulation* (1989) **79**:557–65.

**17.** Ablad B, Bjorkman JA, Gustafsson D et al, The role of sympathetic activity in atherogenesis. Effects of B-blockade, *Am Heart J* (1988) **116**:322–7.

**18.** Winther K, The effect of beta blockade on platelet function and fibrinolytic function, *J Cardiovasc Pharmacol* (1987) **10** (suppl 2):S94–8.

**19.** Roberts R, Modification of infarct size, *Circulation* (1980) **61**:458–9.

**20.** Leading Article, Long-term and short-term beta blockade after myocardial infarction, *Lancet* (1982) **i**:1159–61.

**21.** Hjalmarson A, Elmfledt D, Herlitz J et al, Effect on mortality of metoprolol in acute myocardial infarction, *Lancet* (1981) **ii**:823–7.

**22.** Peter T, Norris RM, Clarke ED et al, Reduction of enzyme levels by propranolol after acute myocardial infarction, *Circulation* (1978) **57**:1091–5.

**23.** Yusuf S, Ramsdale D, Peto R et al, Early intravenous atenolol treatment in suspected acute myocardial infarction. Preliminary report of a randomised trial, *Lancet* (1980) **ii**:273–6.

**24.** Skinner JE, Regulation of cardiac vulnerability by the cerebral defense system, *J Am Coll Cardiol* (1985) **5**:88B–94B.

**25.** Parker GW, Michael LH, Hartley CH, Skinner JE, Entman ML, Central B-adrenergic mechanisms may modulate ischaemic ventricular fibrillation in pigs, *Circulation Research* (1990) **66**:259–70.

**26.** Dellsperger KC, Martins JB, Clothier JL, Marcus ML, Incidence of sudden cardiac death associated with coronary artery occlusion in dogs with hypertension and left ventricular hypertrophy is reduced by chronic B-adrenergic blockade, *Circulation* (1990) **82**:941–50.

**27.** Ablad B, Bjuro T, Bjorkman JA, Edstrom T, Olsson G, Role of central nervous beta-adrenoceptors in the prevention of ventricular fibrillation through augmentation of cardiac vagal tone, *J Am Coll Cardiol* (1991) **17**:165A.

**28.** Olsson G, Tuomilehto J, Berglund G et al, Primary prevention of sudden cardiovascular death in hypertensive patients: mortality results from the MAPHY study, *Am J Hypertens* (1991) **4**:151–8.

**29.** Norwegian Study Group, Timolol-induced reduction in mortality and reinfarction in patients surviving acute myocardial infarction, *N Engl J Med* (1981) **304**:801–7.

**30.** Beta Blocker Heart Attack Trial Research Group, A randomized trial of propranolol in patients with acute myocardial infarction. 1. Mortality results, *JAMA* (1982) **247**:1707–13.

**31.** Ryden L, Ariniego R, Arnman K et al, A double-blind trial of metoprolol in acute myocardial infarction. Effect on ventricular arrhythmias, *N Engl J Med* (1983) **308**:614–18.

**32.** Murray DS, Murray RG, Littler WA, The effects of metoprolol given early in acute myocardial infarction on ventricular arrhythmias, *Eur Heart J* (1986) **7**:217–22.

**33.** Medical Research Council Working Party, MRC trial of treatment of mild hypertension: principal results, *Br Med J* (1985) **59**:364–78.

**34.** Green KG, British MRC trial of treatment for mild hypertension – a more favourable interpretation, *Am J Hypertens* (1991) **4**:723–4.

**35.** The IPPPSH Collaborative Group, Cardiovascular risk and risk factors in a randomized trial of treatment based on the beta-blocker oxprenolol: the International Prospective Primary Prevention Study in Hypertension (IPPPSH), *J Hypertens* (1985) **3**:379–92.

**36.** Wilhelmsen L, Berglund G, Elmfeldt D et al, Beta-blockers versus diuretics in hypertensive men, main results from the HAPPHY trial, *J Hypertens* (1987) **5**:561–72.

**37.** Wikstrand J, Warnold I, Olsson G et al, On behalf of the Advisory Committee. Primary prevention with metoprolol in patients with hypertension. Mortality results from the MAPHY Study, *JAMA* (1988) **259**:1976–82.

**38.** Wikstrand J, Warnold I, Tuomilehto J et al on behalf of the Advisory Committee, Metoprolol versus thiazide diuretics in hypertension. Morbidity results from MAPHY study, *Hypertension* (1991) **17**:579–88.

**39.** Holme I, MAPHY and the two arms of HAPPHY, *JAMA* (1989) **262**:3272–4.

**40.** MRC Working Party, Medical Research Council trial of treatment of hypertension in older adults principal results, *Br Med J* (1992) **304**:405–12.

**41.** Kaplan NM, Critical comments on recent literature: SCRAAPHY about MAPHY from HAPPHY, *Am J Hypertens* (1988) **1:**428–30.

**42.** Moser M, Sheps S, Confusing messages from the newest of the beta blockers/diuretics hypertension trials, *Arch Intern Med* (1989) **149:**2174–5.

**43.** Wikstrand J, Primary prevention in patients with hypertension: comments on the clinical implications of the MAPHY trial, *Am Heart J* (1988) **116:**338–47.

**44.** Wikstrand J, Kendall MJ, The role of beta-blockers in preventing sudden death, *Eur Heart J* (1992) **13** (suppl D):111–20.

**45.** Coope J, Warrender TS, Randomised trial of treatment of hypertension in elderly patients in primary care, *Br Med J* (1986) **293:**1145–51.

**46.** SHEP Cooperative Research Group, Prevention of stroke by antihypertensive drug treatment in older persons with isolated systolic hypertension, *JAMA* (1991) **265:**3255–64.

**47.** Dahlof B, Lindholm LH, Hansson L et al, Morbidity and mortality in the Swedish Trial in old patients with hypertension STOP-Hypertension), *Lancet* (1991) **338:**1281–5.

**48.** Held P, Yusuf S, Early intravenous beta blockade in acute myocardial infarction, *Cardiology* (1989) **76:**132–43.

**49.** ISIS-1 (First International Study of Infarct Survival) Collaborative Group, Mechanisms for the early mortality reduction by beta-blockade started early in acute myocardial infarction, *Lancet* (1988) **i:**921–3.

**50.** The MIAMI Trial Research Group, Metoprolol in Acute Myocardial Infarction (MIAMI), A randomised placebo-controlled international trial, *Eur Heart J* (1985) **6:**199–226.

**51.** Olsson G, Wikstrand J, Warnold I et al, Metoprolol induced reduction in postinfarction mortality: pooled results from five double-blind randomized trials, *Eur Heart J* (1992) **13:**28–32.

**52.** Yusuf S, Peto R, Lewis J, Collins R, Sleight P, Beta blockade during and after myocardial infarction. An overview of the randomized trials, *Prog Cardiovasc Dis* (1985) **27:**335–71.

**53.** The SAVE Investigtors, Effect of captopril on mortality and morbidity in patients with left ventricular dysfunction after myocardial infarcartion, *N Engl J Med* (1992) **327:**669–77.

**54.** The SOLVD Investigators, Effects of enalapril on survival in patients with reduced left ventricular ejection fractions and congestive heart failure, *N Engl J Med* (1991) **325:**293–302.

**55.** The SOLVD Investigators, Effects of enalapril on mortality and the development of heart failure in asymptomatic patients with reduced left ventricular ejection fractions, *N Engl J Med* (1992) **327:**685–91.

**56.** Cohn JN, Johnson G, Zeische S et al (The V-HeFT-II Study), A comparison of enalapril with hydralazine-isosorbide dinitrate in the treatment of chronic congestive heart failure, *N Engl J Med* (1991) **325:**303–10.

**57.** Fonarow GC, Chelimsky-Fallick C, Stevenson LW et al, Effect of direct vasodilation with hydralazine versus angiotensin-converting enzyme inhibition with captopril on mortality in advanced heart failure, The Hy-C trial, *J Am Coll Cardiol* (1992) **19:**842–50.

**58.** Dzau V, Braunwald E, Resolved and unresolved issues in the prevention and treatment of coronary artery disease: a workshop consensus statement, *Am Heart J* (1991) **121:**1244–63.

**59.** Alderman WM, Madhavan S, Ooi WL et al, Association of the renin-sodium profile with the risk of myocardial infarction in patients with hypertension, *N Engl J Med* (1991) **324:**1098–104.

**60.** Bruner HR, Laragh JH, Baer L et al, Essential hypertension: renin and aldosterone, heart attack and stroke, *N Eng J Med* (1972) **286:**441–9.

**61.** Gans ROB, Dunker AJM, Insulin and blood pressure regulation, *J Intern Med* (1991) **229** (suppl 2):49–64.

**62.** Eriksson FK, Lindgarde F, Contributions of estimated insulin resistance and glucose intolerance to essential hypertension, *J Intern Med* (1991) **229** (suppl 2):75–83.

**63.** Berne C, Insulin resistance in hypertension – a relationship with consequences? *J Intern Med* (1991) **229** (suppl 2):65–73.

**64.** Ferriere M, Lachkar H, Richard JL et al, Captopril and insulin sensitivity, *Ann Intern Med* (1985) **102:**134–5.

**65.** Pollare T, Lithell H, Berne C, A comparison of the effects of hydrochlorothiazide and captopril on glucose and lipid metabolism in patients with hypertension, *N Eng J Med* (1989) **321**:868–73.

**66.** Ambrosini E, Bacchelli S, Degli-Esposti D et al, ACE inhibitors and atherosclerosis, *Eur J Epidemiol* (1991) **8** (suppl 1):129–33.

**67.** Dzau VJ, Clinical implications for therapy, possible cardioprotective effects on ACE inhibition, *Br J Clin Pharmacol* (1989) **28**:183S–7S.

**68.** Sharpe N, Murphy J, Smith H et al, Treatment of patients with symptomless left ventricular dysfunction after myocardial infarction, *Lancet* (1988) **i:**255–9.

**69.** Lindpainter K, Jin M, Wilhelm MJ et al, Intercardiac generation of angiotensin and its physiologic role, *Circulation* (1988) **77**: I-18–I-24.

**70.** Ertl G, Bauer B, Gaudron P et al, Possibilities of ACE inhibition therapy in acute myocardial ischaemia, *Klin-wochenschr* (1991) **69** (suppl 24):10–17.

**71.** McMurray J, Chopra M, Influence of ACE inhibitors on free radicals and reperfusion injury: pharmacological curiosity or therapeutic hope? *Br J Clin Pharmacol* (1991) **31**:373–9.

**72.** Chopra M, Beswick H, Clapperton M et al, Antioxidant effects of angiotensin-converting enzyme (ACE) inhibitors, free radical and oxidant scavenging are sulfhydryl dependent, bulipid peroxidation is inhibited by both sulfhydryl and nonsulfhydryl-containing ACE inhibitors, *J Cardiovasc Pharmacol* (1991) **19**:330–40.

**73.** Packer M, Lee WH, Kessler PD et al, Role of neurohormonal mechanisms in determining survival in patients with severe chronic heart failure, *Circulation* (1987) **75** (suppl iv): iv80–iv91.

**74.** The CAPPP Group, The Captopril prevention project: a prospective intervention trial of angiotensin converting enzyme inhibitor in the treatment of hypertension, *J Hypertens* (1990) **8**:985–90.

**75.** The CONSENSUS Trial Study Group, Effects of enalapril on mortality in severe congestive heart failure: results of the Cooperative North Scandinavian Enalapril Survival Study (CONSENSUS), *N Engl J Med* (1987) **316**:1429–35.

**76.** Oldroyd KG, Pye M, Ray SG et al, Effects of early captopril administration on infarct expansion, left ventricular remodelling and exercise capacity after acute myocardial infarction, *Am J Cardiol* (1991) **68**:713–18.

**77.** The CONSENSUS II Study Group, Effects of the early administration of enalapril on mortality in patients with acute myocardial infarction. Results of the Cooperative New Scandinavian Enalapril Survival Study II (CONSENSUS II), *N Engl J Med* (1992) **327**:678–84.

**78.** Sharpe N, Smith H, Murphy J et al, Early prevention of left ventricular dysfunction after myocardial infarction with angiotensin-converting enzyme inhibition, *Lancet* (1991) **337**:872–6.

**79.** Pfeffer MA, Lamas GA, Vaughan MD et al, Effect of captopril on progressive ventricular dilatation after interior myocardial infarction, *N Engl J Med* (1988) **319**:80–6.

**80.** Kleber FX, Niemoller L, Doering W, Impact of converting enzyme inhibition on progression of chronic heart failure: results of the Munich Mild Heart Failure Trial, *Br Heart J* (1992) **67**:289–96.

**81.** Henry, PD, Atherogenesis, calcium and calcium antagonist, *Am J Cardiol* (1990) **66**:3-I-6-I.

**82.** Venkata C, Ram S, Anti-atherosclerotic and vasculoprotective actions of calcium antagonists, *Am J Cardiol* (1990) **66**:29–32.

**83.** Fleckenstein-Grun G, Frey M, Thimm F et al, Differentiation between calcium and cholesterol-dominated types of arteriosclerotic lesions: antiarteriosclerotic aspects of calcium antagonists, *J Cardiovasc Pharmacol* (1991) **18** (Suppl 6): S1–9.

**84.** Fleckenstein-Grun G, Frey M, Thimm F et al, A calcium overload – an important cellular mechanism in hypertension and arteriosclerosis, *Drugs* (1992) **44** (suppl 1):23–30.

**85.** Keogh A, Schroeder JS, A review of calcium antagonists and atherosclerosis, *J Cardiovasc Pharmacol* (1990) **16** (suppl 6): S28–35.

**86.** Schneider W, Kober G, Roebruck P et al, Retardation of development and progression of coronary atherosclerosis: a new indication for calcium antagonists? *Eur J Clin Pharmacol* (1990) **39** (suppl1):S17–23.

**87.** Parmley W, Vascular protection from atherosclerosis: potential of calcium antagonists, *Am J Cardiol* (1990) **66**:16–22.

**88.** Dale J, Landmark KH, Myhre E, The effects of nifedipine, a calcium antagonist on platelet function, *Am Heart J* (1983) **105**:103–5.

**89.** Ferrari R, Visioli O, Protective effects of calcium antagonists against ischaemic and reperfusion damage, *Drugs* (1991) **42** (suppl 1):14–27.

**90.** Nayler WG, Basic mechanisms involved in the protection of the ischaemic myocardium: the role of calcium antagonists, *Drugs* (1991) **42**(suppl 2):21–7.

**91.** Skolnick AE, Frishman WH, Calcium channel blockers in myocardial infarction, *Arch Intern Med* (1989) **149**:1669–77.

**92.** Loaldi A, Polese A, Montorsi P et al, Comparison of nifedipine, propranolol and ISDN on angiographic progression and regression of coronary arterial narrowings in angina pectoris, *Am J Cardiol* (1989) **64**:433–9.

**93.** The INTACT Study Group, Retardation of angiographic progression of coronary disease with nifedipine. Results of INTACT, *Lancet* (1990) **335**:3–7.

**94.** Waters D, Lesperance J, Francetich M et al, A controlled clinical trial to assess the effect of calcium antagonist upon the progression of coronary atherosclerosis, *Circulation* (1990) **82**:1940–53.

**95.** Sirnes PA, Overskeid K, Pedersen TR et al, Evaluation of infarct size during the early use of nifedipine in patients with acute myocardial infarction: the Norwegian Nifedipine Multicentre Trial, *Cirulation* (1984) **70**:638–44.

**96.** Muller JE, Morrison J, Stone PH et al, Nifedipine therapy for patients with threatened and acute myocardial infarction: a randomised double blind, placebo controlled comparison, *Circulation* (1984) **69**:740–7.

**97.** Wilcox RG, Hampton JR, Banks DC et al, Trial of early nifedipine in acute myocardial infarction: the TRENT Study, *Br Med J* (1986) **293**:1204–7.

**98.** Branagan JP, Walsh K, Kelly P et al, Effect of early treatment with nifedipine in suspected acute myocardial infarction, *Eur Heart J* (1986) **7**:859–65.

**99.** Erbel R, Pop T, Meinertz T et al, Combination of calcium channel blocker and thrombolytic therapy in acute myocardial infarction, *Am Heart J* (1988) **115**:529–38.

**100.** Report of the Holland Interuniversity Nifedipine/Metoprolol Trial (HINT) Research Group, Early treatment of unstable angina in the coronary care unit: a randomised, double blind, placebo controlled comparison of recurrent ischaemia in patients treated with nifedipine or metoprolol or both, *Br Heart J* (1986) **56**:400–13.

**101.** Walker L, MacKenzie G, Adgey J, Effect of nifedipine in the early phase of acute myocardial infarction on enzymatically estimated infarct size and arrhythmias, *Br Heart J* (1987) **57**:83–4.

**102.** Gottileb SO, Becker LC, Weiss JL et al, Nifedipine in acute myocardial infarction: an assessment of left ventricular function, infarct size and infarct expansion. A double blind, randomised, placebo controlled trial, *Br Heart J* (1988) **59**:411–18.

**103.** Israeli SPRINT Study Group, Secondary prevention reinfarction Israeli nifedipine trial (SPRINT). A randomised intervention trial of nifedipine in patients with acute myocardial infarction, *Eur Heart J* (1988) **9**:354–64.

**104.** SPRINT Study Group, Secondary prevention re-infarction Israeli nifedipine trial (SPRINT II), *Eur Heart J* (1988) **9** (suppl 1):350.

**105.** Held PH, Yusuf S, Furberg CD, Calcium channel blockers in acute myocardial infarction and unstable angina: an overview, *Br Med J* (1989) **299**:1187–92.

**106.** Midtbo KA, Effects of long term verapamil therapy on serum lipids and other metabolic parameters, *Am J Cardiol* (1990) **66**:13-I–15-I.

**107.** Kober G, Schneider W, Kaltenback M. Can the progression of coronary sclerosis be influenced by calcium antagonists? *J Cardiovasc Pharmacol* (1989) **13**(suppl 4):S2–6.

**108.** Magnani B, Dal-Palu C, Zanchetti A (Verapamil in Hypertension Atherosclerosis Study Investigators), Preliminary clinical experience with calcium antagonists in atherosclerosis, *Drugs* (1992) **44** (suppl 1): 128–33.

**109.** Crea F, Deanfield J, Crean P et al, Effects of verapamil in preventing early postinfarction angina and reinfarction, *Am J Cardiol* (1985) **55**:900–4.

110. Bussman WD, Seher W, Gruengras M, Reduction of creatinine kinase and creatinine kinase-MB indexes of infarct size by intravenous verapamil, *Am J Cardiol* (1984) **54**:1224–30.

111. Danish Study Group on Verapamil in Myocardial Infarction, The Danish studies on verapamil in myocardial infarction, *Br J Clin Pharm* (1986) **21**:197S–204S.

112. Danish Study Group on Verapamil in Myocardial Infarction, The effect of verapamil on mortality and major events after acute myocardial infarction. The Danish Verapamil Infarction Trial II (DAVIT II), *Am J Cardiol* (1990) **66**:779–85.

113. Gibson RS, Boden WE, Theroux P et al, Diltiazem and reinfarction in patients with non Q wave myocardial infarction: results of a double blind randomized multicentre trial, *N Engl J Med* (1986) **315**:423–9.

114. Zannad F, Amor M, Karcher G et al, Effect of diltiazem on myocardial infarct size estimated by enzyme release, serial thallium-201 single-photon emission computed tomography and radionuclide angiography, *Am J Cardiol* (1988) **61**:1172–7.

115. The Multicentre Diltiazem Post-Infarction Trial Research Group, The effect of diltiazem on mortality and reinfarction after myocardial infarction, *N Engl J Med* (1988) **319**:385–92.

116. Boden WE, Krone RJ, Kleiger RE et al, Diltiazem reduces long-term cardiac event rate after non-Q-wave infarction: Multicentre Diltiazem Post Infarction Trial (MDPIT), *Circulation* (1988) **78** (suppl 2):II-96 (Abstract).

117. Consensus Conference, Lowering blood cholesterol to prevent heart disease, *JAMA* (1985) **253**:2080–6.

118. Leren P, Comparison of effects on lipid metabolism of antihypertensive drugs with alpha and beta adrenergic antagonist properties, *Am J Med* (1987) **82** (suppl 1A):31–5.

119. Kincaid–Smith P, Alpha$_1$–blockers, their antihypertensive efficacy and effects on lipids and lipoprotein, *J Hum Hypertens* (1989) **3**(suppl 2):75–83.

120. Grimm R, Thiazide diuretics and selective alpha blockers: comparison of use in antihypertensive therapy including possible differences in coronary heart disease risk reduction, *Am J Med* (1987) **82**(suppl 1A): 26–30.

121. Leren P, Foss PO, Helgeland A et al, Effects of propranolol and prazosin on blood lipids, *Lancet* (1980) **ii**:4–6.

122. Lowenstein J, Neusy AJ, Effects of prazosin and propranolol on serum lipids in patients with essential hypertension, *Am J Med* (1984) **76**(suppl 2A):79–84.

123. Rouffy J, Jaillard J, Effects of two antihypertensive agents on lipids, lipoproteins A and B, *Am J Med* (1986) **80**(suppl 2A):100–3.

124. Krone W, Nagele J, Metabolic changes during antihypertensive therapies, *J Hum Hypertens* (1989) **3**(suppl 2):69–74.

125. Frick MH, Halttunen P, Himanen P et al, A long term double blind comparison of doxazosin and atenolol in patients with mild to moderate essential hypertension, *Br J Clin Pharmacol* (1986) **21**:55S–62S.

126. Castrignano R, D'Angelo A, Pati T et al, A single–blind study of doxazosin in the treatment of mild-to-moderate essential hypertensive patients with concomitant noninsulin-dependent diabetes mellitus, *Am Heart J* (1988) **116**:1778–84.

127. Lehtonen A and Finnish Multicentre Study Group, Lowered levels of serum insulin, glucose and cholesterol in hypertensive patients during treatment with doxazosin, *Curr Ther Res* (1990) **121**:251–60.

128. Feher MD, Henderson AD, Wadsworth J et al, Alpha-blocker therapy; a possible advance in the treatment of diabetic hypertension – results of a cross-over study of doxazosin and atenolol monotherapy in hypertensive non-insulin dependent diabetic subjects, *J Hum Hypertens* (1990) **4**:571–77.

129. Leren P, The cardiovascular effects of alpha-receptor blocking agents, *J Hypertens* (1992) **10** (suppl 3):S11–14.

130. Bell FP, Effects of antihypertensive agents propranolol, metoprolol, nadolol, prazosin and chlortalidone on LCAT activity in rabbit and rat aortas and in LCAT activity in human plasma in vitro, *J Cardiovasc Pharmacol* (1985) **7**:437–42.

131. Leren TP, Doxazosin low-density lipoprotein receptor activity, *Acta Pharmacol Toxicol* (1985) **56**:269–72.

132. Krone W, Muller-Wieland D, Nagele H et al, Effects of adrenergic antihypertensives and Ca$^{++}$ on LDL receptor synthesis in

human mononuclear leukocytes, *Arteriosclerosis* (1985) **5**:542a.

**133.** Ferrannini E, Buzzigoli G, Bonadonna R et al, Insulin resistance in essential hypertension, *N Engl J Med* (1987) **317**:350–7.

**134.** Pollare T, Lithell H, Selinus I et al, Application of prazosin is associated with an increase of insulin sensitivity in obese patients with hypertension, *Diabetologia* (1988) **31**:415–20.

**135.** Lehtonen A and the Finnish Multicentre Study Group, Doxazosin effects on the insulin and glucose in hypertensive patients, *Am Heart J* (1991) **121**:1307–11.

**136.** Leenen FH, Smith DL, Farkas RM et al, Vasodilators and regression of left ventricular hypertrophy. Hydralazine versus prazosin in hypertensive humans, *Am J Med* (1987) **82**:969–78.

**137.** Agabiti-Rosei E, Muiesan ML, Rizzoni D et al, Reduction of left ventricular hypertrophy after long term antihypertensive treatment with doxazosin, *J Hum Hypertens* (1992) **6**:9–15.

**138.** Yasumoto K, Takata M, Toshida K et al, Reversal of left ventricular hypertrophy by terazosin in hypertensive patients, *J Hum Hypertens* (1990) **4**:13–18.

**139.** Hernandez RH, Carvajal AR, Pajuelo JG et al, The effect of doxazosin on platelet aggregation in normotensive subjects and patients with hypertension: An in vitro study, *Am Heart J* (1991) **121**:389–94.

**140.** Jansson JH, Johansson B, Boman K et al, Effects of doxazosin and atenolol on the fibrinolytic system in patients with hypertension and elevated serum cholesterol, *Eur J Clin Pharmacol* (1991) **40**:321–6.

**141.** Lytle TB, Coles SJ, Waite MA, A multicentre hospital study of the efficacy and safety of terazosin and its effects on the plasma cholesterol levels of patients with essential hypertension, *J Clin Pharmacol Ther* (1991) **16**:263–73.

**142.** Stamler J, Prineas RJ, Neaton JD et al, Background and design of the New US trial on diet and drug treatment of mild hypertension (TOMHS), *Am J Cardiol* (1987) **59**:51G–60G.

**143.** Furberg CD, Yusuf S, Effects of drug therapy on survival in chronic congestive heart failure, *Am J Cardiol* (1988) **62**:41A–45A.

**144.** Murrell W. Nitroglycerine as a remedy for angina pectoris, *Lancet* (1879) **i**: 80,113,151,225.

**145.** Kendall MJ, Long term therapeutic efficacy with once-daily isosorbide-5-mononitrate (Imdur), *J Clin Pharmacol Ther* (1990) **15**:169–85.

**146.** Olsson G, Allgen J. Prophylactic nitrate therapy in angina pectoris: possibilities to optimise treatment, *Can J Cardiol* (1993) **9**(suppl A):1A–5A.

**147.** Yusuf S, Collins R, MacMahon S et al, Effect of intravenous nitrates on mortality in acute myocardial infarctions: an overview of the randomised trials, *Lancet* (1988) **ii**:1088–92.

**148.** ISIS-4 Collaborative Group, Fourth International Study of Infarct Survival: protocol for a large simple study of the effects of oral mononitrate, of oral captopril and of intravenous magnesium *Am J Cardiol* (1991) **68**:87D–100D.

**149.** Abrams J, Hemodynamic effects of nitroglycerin and long acting nitrates, *Am Heart J* (1985) **110**:216–24.

**150.** Jugdutt BI, Role of nitrates after acute myocardial infarction, *Am J. Cardiol* (1992) **70**:82B–87B.

**151.** Abrams J, Mechanisms of action of the organic nitrates in the treatment of myocardial ischaemia, *Am J Cardiol* (1992) **70**:30B–42B.

**152.** Yeung AC, Vekshtein VI, Krantz DS et al, The effects of atherosclerosis on the vasomotor response of coronary arteries to mental stress, *N Engl J Med* (1991) **325**:1551–6.

**153.** Lam JYT, Chesebro JH, Fuster V, Platelets, vasoconstriction and nitroglycerin during arterial wall injury, *Circulation* (1988) **78**:712–16.

**154.** Johnstone M, Lam JYT, Waters D, The antithrombotic action of nitroglycerin: cyclic GMP as a potential mediator, *J Am Coll Cardiol* (1989) **13**:231 (abstract).

**155.** Diodati J, Theroux P, Latour JG et al, Effects of nitroglycerin at therapeutic doses on platelet aggregation in unstable angina pectoris and acute myocardial infarction, *Am J Cardiol* (1990) **66**:683–8.

**156.** Tofler GH, Brezinski D, Schufer AI et al, Concurrent morning increase in platelet aggregability and the risk of myocardial infarction and sudden cardiac death, *N Engl J Med* (1987) **316**:1514–19.

**157.** Mulcahy D, Keegan J, Cunningham D et al, Circadian variation of total ischaemic burden and its alteration with anti-anginal agents. *Lancet* (1988) **ii**:755–8.

**158.** Jugdutt BI, Warnica JW, Intravenous nitroglycerin therapy to limit myocardial infarct size, expansion and complications: effect of timing, dosage and infarct location, *Circulation* (1988) **78**:906–19.

**159.** Humen D, McCormick L, Jugdutt BI, Chronic reduction of left ventricular volumes at rest and exercise in patients treated with nitroglycerin following anterior myocardial infarction, *J Am Coll Cardiol* (1989) **13**:25A.

**160.** Flaherty JT, Come PC, Baird MG et al, Effects of intravenous nitro-glycerin on left ventricular function and ST segment changes in acute myocardial infarction, *Br Heart J* (1976) **38**:612–21.

**161.** Bussman WD, Passek D, Seidal W et al, Reduction of CK and CK-MB indexes of infarct size by intravenous nitroglycerin, *Circulation* (1981) **63**:615–22.

**162.** Jaffe AS, Geltman EM, Tiefenbrum AJ et al, Relation of the extent of inferior myocardial infarction with intravenous nitroglycerin: a randomised prospective study, *Br Heart J* (1983) **49**:452–60.

**163.** Derrida JR, Sal R, Chiche P, Effects of prolonged nitroglycerin infusion in patients with acute myocardial infarction, *Am J Cardiol* (1978) **41**:407 (abstract).

**164.** Chiarello M, Gold HK, Leinback RC et al, Comparison between the effects of nitroprusside and nitroglycerin on ischaemic injury during acute myocardial infarction, *Circulation* (1976) **54**:766–73.

**165.** Mann T, Cohn PH, Holman BL et al, Effects of nitroprusside on regional myocardial blood flow in coronary disease: results in 25 patients and comparison with nitroglycerin, *Circulation* (1978) **57**:732–8.

# Chapter 3
# **Hyperlipidaemia**

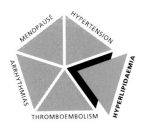

If one takes at face value the story of an 88-year-old man who ate up to 30 eggs each day and yet survived without developing any signs of atherosclerosis[1] – no history of myocardial ischaemia, stroke or renal disease – one might suppose that the notion of cholesterol as an important determinant of cardiovascular disease was less than secure. Bedevilled by controversy, the cholesterol hypothesis of coronary heart disease has become almost a parody within clinical science. Trials are discussed and reinterpreted endlessly; there is an abundance of opinion, to which we are now contributing. The data can be used to fit just about any argument either in favour of or against cholesterol. Examine one recent analysis by Petr Skrabanek:[2]

> Despite the fact that the cholesterol and fats in the diet represent only one of about 300 risk factors for coronary heart disease, dietary cholesterol has been portrayed by many experts as the archvillain. . . . Of the many different kinds of evidence used in support of [this] hypothesis, only randomised, controlled trials of intervention are of practical relevance. These trials have failed to demonstrate benefit . . . .

Contrast his scepticism with the certainty expressed by others:[3]

> . . . the clinical studies performed to date provide unequivocal evidence that modification of the serum lipoproteins substantially protects against coronary heart disease.

One must obviously tread with extreme care when assessing the evidence that lies between these two opposing points of view. Yet such explicit disagreements can be rationalized and the question of cardioprotection can be answered, although the *overall benefit* to the patient of reducing serum cholesterol remains unresolved.

But before we discuss the cardioprotective efficacy of lipid-lowering therapies, we must briefly orientate ourselves concerning lipid and lipoprotein metabolism and theories of atherogenesis.

# ■ LIPID AND LIPOPROTEIN METABOLISM

Cholesterol was first isolated from a biliary calculus in 1769 by Poulletier de la Salle. In 1896, Hurthle discovered cholesteryl esters in blood. During the ensuing century, it has become clear that, since cholesterol, triglycerides and phospholipids are insoluble in water, their transport in blood can only be achieved by combination with protein. Four main classes of lipoprotein are recognized (Table 3.1).[4] Moreover, lipoproteins are dynamic structures with constantly varying composition. Some of their important differences in protein constituents are shown in Table 3.2.

|  | Density (g/ml) | Mean diameter (nm) | Electrophoretic mobility |
| --- | --- | --- | --- |
| Chylomicrons | <0.95 | 100–1000 | Origin |
| VLDL | <1.006 | 43 | pre-β |
| IDL | 1.006–1.019 | 27 | β |
| LDL | 1.019–1.063 | 22 | β |
| HDL$_2$ | 1.06–1.125 | 9.5 | α |
| HDL$_3$ | 1.125–1.21 | 6.5 | α |
| Lp(a) | 1.05?–1.082 | 26 | pre-β$_1$ |

**Table 3.1** Properties of plasma lipoproteins.

## □ Apoproteins

Apoproteins are the protective components of lipoproteins and serve three main functions. First, they solubilize cholesterol esters and triglyceride; second, they influence the interaction of these lipids with enzymes such as LCAT (lecithin:cholesterol acyltransferase), lipoprotein lipase and hepatic lipase; and third, they bind to specific cell surface receptors.[6]

| | Chylo-microns | VLDL | LDL | HDL | Chromo-some |
|---|---|---|---|---|---|
| **Total protein (mg/dl plasma)** | | | | | |
| | – | 6 | 80 | 190 | |
| **Aproproteins (% total protein)** | | | | | |
| Apo AI | Trace | Trace | Trace | 66 | 11 |
| Apo AII | Trace | Trace | Trace | 20 | 1 |
| Apo B | 5–20 | 37 | 97 | – | 2 |
| Apo CI | 15 | 3 | Trace | 3 | 19 |
| Apo CII | 15 | 7 | Trace | Trace | 19 |
| Apo CIII | 40–50 | 40 | 2 | 4 | 11 |
| Apo D | – | – | – | 5 | 3 |
| Apo E | 4 | 13 | 1 | 1 | 19 |

**Table 3.2** Protein composition of lipoproteins in fasting plasma.[5]

Apo A is the main protein component of high-density lipoprotein (HDL). Apo AI activates LCAT and apo AII activates hepatic lipase.

Apo B (B for bad is a helpful reminder) is composed of two main types: apo $B_{100}$ and apo $B_{48}$. Apo $B_{100}$ is found in chylomicrons, very low density lipoprotein (VLDL) and low-density lipoprotein (LDL); apo $B_{48}$ is found in chylomicrons only. Apo $B_{48}$ is produced in the intestine and represents the N-terminal portion of apo $B_{100}$, while the latter is an LDL receptor ligand. Apo $B_{100}$ is produced in the liver. Lipoproteins contain only one apo B molecule per particle.

Apo C is a major constituent of VLDL. Apo CI activates LCAT and apo CII activates lipoprotein lipase; there is also an apo CIII. The function of apo D is unknown, although it may have a role in cholesteryl ester transfer. Apo E is polymorphic and is involved in cholesterol transfer between tissues. Apolipoproteins F, G and H have also been characterized.

# ☐ Lipoproteins

Chylomicrons are the largest lipid particles and are responsible for transporting dietary triglyceride (90 per cent of their mass) from the intestine to the systemic circulation. Their half-life is less than 1 h and they are normally undetectable after a 12-h fast. Peak plasma concentrations are reached 3–6 h after eating a meal. As triglyceride is gradually removed, the apoprotein constituents alter such that chylomicron remnants retain apo $B_{48}$ and apo E; apo E then binds to the hepatocyte chylomicron remnant receptor that clears remnants from the circulation.

VLDL is synthesized in the liver and intestine and its main function is to transport triglyceride. VLDL particles contain relatively more cholesteryl ester than chylomicrons. Loss of triglyceride converts VLDL into IDL (intermediate-density lipoprotein, also known as LDL, or VLDL remnant); IDL is either removed by the liver or converted into $LDL_2$.

LDL contains one molecule of apo $B_{100}$ per particle and transports 75 per cent of total plasma cholesterol. It carries cholesteryl ester to tissues and returns the excess to the liver for excretion.

HDL is divided into three classes: $HDL_1$, $HDL_2$, and $HDL_3$ (depending on ultracentrifugation characteristics). Synthesized in the liver and intestine, HDL plays a key part in mobilizing tissue cholesterol.

Lp(a) consists of one LDL particle covalently linked to one molecule of apolipoprotein (a). Lp(a) shares substantial sequence homology with plasminogen, which contains five cysteine-rich structures called kringles. These are involved in binding fibrin, and apo(a) has a long sequence of kringle-4 subunits. However, the exciting possibility of a link between atherogenesis and thrombogenesis – centred around the Lp(a) particle – might be spurious since kringle-4 domains lack the arginine residues that are necessary for fibrin binding and the apo(a) molecule lacks the proteolytic cleavage site necessary for the enzymic activity of plasminogen.

A simplified scheme for lipoprotein metabolism is shown in Figure 3.1.

Apart from key regulatory enzymes (hepatic and lipoprotein lipase, LCAT), together with lipid-transfer proteins (such as cholesterol-ester-transfer protein), two key points in lipid metabolism merit further attention: the LDL receptor and HMG-CoA reductase.

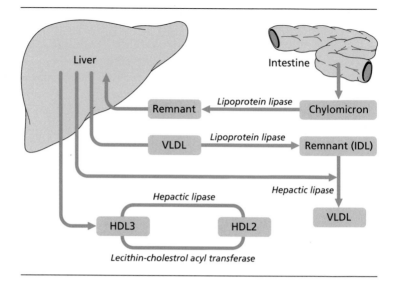

**Figure 3.1** A simplified approach to lipoprotein metabolism. LPL = lipoprotein lipase; HL = hepatic lipase; LCAT = lecithin:cholesterol acyltransferase.

The discovery of the LDL receptor led to Nobel prizes being given to Brown and Goldstein in 1985.[7] LDL receptors are found clustered together on the surface of cells in clathrin-coated pits. LDL binding leads to internalization of LDL–receptor complexes, return of receptors to the cell surface, and finally catabolism of LDL particles by lysosomal enzymes. These receptors bind both apo $B_{100}$ and apo E and remove 75 per cent of LDL. The gene for the LDL receptor is located on chromosome 19; mutations to this gene lead to impaired clearance of LDL and hence familial hypercholesterolaemia (FH).

Free intracellular cholesterol that is liberated then controls the rate of cholesterol synthesis by downregulating the enzyme HMG-CoA reductase. This enzyme is found mainly in the liver, small intestine, adrenal glands and gonads. 3-Hydroxy-3-methylglutaryl-CoA is converted to mevalonic acid and thence to cholesterol, which subsequently downregulates the enzyme's activity. Drugs that inhibit HMG-CoA reductase prevent cholesterol synthesis and enhance receptor-mediated LDL uptake, thus lowering circulating concentrations of cholesterol.

# ■ THE CHOLESTEROL HYPOTHESIS

Although there is debate about the management of hyperlipidaemic patients, the evidence for a causal link between hypercholesterolaemia and atheroma formation is well established.

## □ Biological evidence

Atherogenesis involves two main processes: endothelial/intimal damage to the luminal surface of the vessel wall and focal accumulation of cellular and acellular components leading to disruption of the media. Four main factors influence rates of atherosclerosis: age, sex, plasma cholesterol and blood pressure.

The characteristic lesion of atheroma is the fibrous plaque, a mass of smooth muscle cells and fibrous tissue surrounding a core of lipid, which is covered by endothelium. The cholesterol in the lesion is derived mostly from the blood. The importance of plasma cholesterol is emphasized by the severity of the disease process in those with FH, where LDL concentrations are over twice normal. Moreover, partial ileal bypass, which mobilizes large quantities of tissue cholesterol, leads to substantial regression of coronary atheromatous lesions demonstrable by angiography.

Endothelial damage is central to the process of atheroma formation.[8] Injury (excessively high blood pressure or hypercholesterolaemia) leads to the binding of platelets to the arterial wall, which triggers medial smooth muscle cell proliferation (via platelet-derived growth factor) and subsequently smooth muscle cell migration into the media.[9] In addition, in the presence of high circulating concentrations of cholesterol, monocytes bind to the vessel wall, penetrate the endothelium, accumulate lipid, and become foam cells (once thought to be derived from smooth muscle cells).[10]

The endothelium overlying these foam cells appears as fatty streaks and is eventually disrupted, exposing underlying tissue. Platelets adhere, a thrombosis develops, and smooth muscle proliferation proceeds apace with the fatty streak becoming a proliferative lesion.

The cholesterol-laden foam cell (formerly a monocyte, which on entering the tissue becomes a macrophage) is the most notable feature of the fibrous plaque. Intuitively, one would guess that macrophages acquire cholesteryl ester from the high circulating concentrations of LDL. However, once cholesterol in a macrophage begins to accumulate, its LDL receptors become downregulated, thus switching off further cholesterol uptake. This might be expected to prevent cholesterol accumulation but does not always do so.

This paradox might be explained by oxidized LDL. LDL phospholipids become oxidized in vitro in the presence of macrophages, smooth muscle cells and endothelial cells.[11] This process is enhanced by LDL particles that are rich in polyunsaturated fatty acids. Oxidized LDL is then taken up by macrophages via another receptor subtype: the acetyl-LDL receptor.[12] Acetyl-LDL receptors on the macrophage surface do not downregulate. There is also now substantial evidence that oxidized LDL exists in vivo.[3]

Evidence supporting a causal role for cholesterol in atheroma formation also comes from animal models in which diet-induced hypercholesterolaemia leads to reversible atheroma formation.[13] In humans, angiographic data also support the cholesterol hypothesis. Angiographic abnormalities can be correlated with the degree of hypercholesterolaemia, more specifically with increased LDL and decreased HDL concentrations. For example, moderate reductions in LDL cholesterol (from 5.7 to 4.6 mmol/l) by treatment with cholestyramine lead to a significant reduction in the number of coronary lesions that progress.[14] In the Cholesterol Lowering Atherosclerosis Study, treatment with colestipol and nicotinic acid reduced LDL cholesterol from 4.1 to 2.5 mmol/l and led to a significant increase in lesion regression[15] (Figure 3.2). Both of these studies were double-blind and provide strong direct evidence for the causal role of cholesterol in atherogenesis.

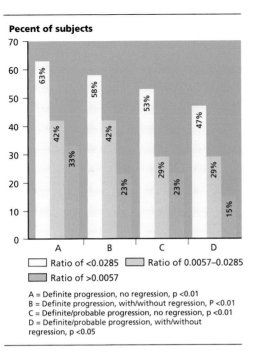

**Pecent of subjects**

Legend:
☐ Ratio of <0.0285   ☐ Ratio of 0.0057–0.0285
■ Ratio of >0.0057

A = Definite progression, no regression, p <0.01
B = Definite progression, with/without regression, P <0.01
C = Definite/probable progression, no regression, p <0.01
D = Definite/probable progression, with/without
regression, p <0.05

**Figure 3.2** Relation between HDL cholesterol/total cholesterol ratio and coronary artery disease progression. A = definite progression, no regression, $p < 0.01$; B = definite progression, with/without regression, $p < 0.01$; C = definite/probable progression, no regression, $p < 0.01$; D = definite/probable progression, with/without regression, $p < 0.05$.[15]

Additional (perhaps the best) evidence that LDL is athero-genic also comes from work on FH.[3] The gene for the LDL receptor in FH is either deficient or absent. High circulating LDL concentrations in both heterozygous and homozygous subjects lead to accelerated atherosclerosis, more so in those who are homozygous.

## ☐ Epidemiological evidence

Three lines of epidemiological data point to a relation between hypercholesterolaemia and coronary artery disease (CAD).

First, there is a close correlation between the incidence of ischaemic heart disease among middle-aged men (40–59 years old) and the proportion whose serum cholesterol exceeds 6.5 mmol/l.[16] The seven countries studied revealed that differences in serum cholesterol between countries were largely attributable to differences in dietary saturated fat intake. This report has been severely criticized for biased sample selection (only 499 of the total 12 770 male participants had detailed dietary surveys taken) and inconsistent and non-standardized data collection.[17]

Second, case-control studies have suggested that those who develop coronary heart disease have increased concentrations of circulating lipids compared with those who have no coronary heart disease.[18] These studies might also be subject to bias and the only truly reliable evidence comes from prospective surveys.

The best known prospective study comes from Framingham and began in 1949 with over 5000 participants. The investigators found that CAD was strikingly increased among those who smoked or who had hypercholesterolaemia or hypertension.[19] Furthermore, the Multiple Risk Factor Intervention Trial showed that the risk attributable to cholesterol was continuous over the whole range of serum cholesterol concentrations.[20] The risk of CAD rose substantially when the serum cholesterol exceeded 6.5 mmol/l: a death rate of over 12 per 1000 men compared with a rate of below 6 per 1000 men if serum cholesterol was below 5.2 mmol/l.

Most of the cholesterol risk resides in the LDL particle and apo B measurements are a convenient marker of circulating LDL since there is a 1 : 1 ratio of apo B to LDL. Case-control studies[21] support the value of apo B measurements in determining risk for future CAD.

The protective effect of HDL for coronary heart disease was also convincingly shown in the Framingham study.[22] HDL is probably beneficial by means of reverse cholesterol transport from tissues back to the liver or by preventing thrombus formation in some, as yet, poorly defined way. Just as apo B is a better discriminating marker for risk than LDL or serum cholesterol, so apo AI (A for acceptable) is likely to be a better and more reliable measure than HDL. At present, however, various ratios – HDL/LDL, for example – are used to estimate the balance of risk between HDL and LDL particles.

More recent evidence points to the value of HDL in predicting coronary heart disease. Romm and colleagues[23] found that HDL cholesterol was the most powerful independent variable associated with the presence and severity of CAD among 197 patients undergoing diagnostic coronary angiography. The value of the total/HDL cholesterol ratio in women as an indicator of the presence, severity and extent of CAD has also been confirmed.[24] The importance of $HDL_2$ versus $HDL_3$ is still a matter of debate. Some believe that $HDL_2$ is the key particle that confers risk reduction,[25] while others have shown independent correlations with risk for $HDL_3$.[26]

The influence of triglycerides remains controversial and is complex.[27]

High concentrations of Lp(a) are also associated with coronary heart disease, but whether this risk is independent of high LDL remains unknown. In cross-sectional studies, Lobo and colleagues have shown that Lp(a) is an independent risk factor for cardiovascular disease.[28]

Whatever one's quibbles with individual studies (and there are many; few reports achieve the purist's demands of perfection), a substantial body of evidence supports the notion that cholesterol is a necessary and, in some cases although not all, sufficient factor for atheroma formation. There are clearly enough data to support an *a priori* hypothesis that reducing cholesterol will be cardioprotective.

## ☐ Therapeutic evidence

Three major clinical trials have documented the clinical effects of reducing plasma lipids. In the Lipid Research Clinics Program,[29] patients were treated with cholestyramine; in the Helsinki Heart Study,[30] Gemfibrozil was given; and in the Coronary Drug Project,[31] niacin was used.

The Lipid Research Clinics Coronary Prevention Trial enrolled 3806 middle-aged symptom-free men. They were randomized to receive cholestyramine 24 g (six sachets) daily or placebo for an average of 7.4 years. The mean plasma total cholesterol on diet at entry was 280.4 mg/dl (7.25 mmol/l), at 1 year was 238.6 mg/dl (6.17 mmol/l), and after 7 years was 257.1 mg/dl (6.65 mmol/l). The hyperlipidaemia was therefore not severe, cholesterol reduction was modest, and compliance was poor. Nevertheless the incidence of definite coronary deaths and definite myocardial infarctions (MIs) was reduced from 189 (9.8 per cent) on placebo to 155 (8.1 per cent) on cholestyramine ($p = 0.05$). Total mortality rates – 3.7 and 3.6 per cent – were not different.

The Coronary Drug Project originally recruited 8341 men who had had an ECG-documented MI. They were randomized to several treatment options, three of which were stopped because of unacceptable adverse effects. However, 1119 men were randomized to receive niacin and 2789 took placebo. Follow-up was continued for 15 years, at which point niacin therapy was shown to be associated with an 11 per cent reduction in total mortality (52 per cent versus 58 per cent, $p = 0.0004$). Treatment reduced serum cholesterol concentrations by 10.1 per cent; the impact on mortality was greatest in those whose cholesterol was over 250 mg/dl (6.5 mmol/l).

The Helsinki Heart Study was a double-blind randomized 5-year trial of gemfibrozil in 4081 symptom-free men with a cholesterol of 270 mg/dl (7 mmol/l), which fell to 247 mg/dl (6.4 mmol/l). HDL was increased and LDL was reduced. Deaths per 1000 patients from ischaemic heart disease were reduced from 9.4 to 6.8, though total mortality – 21.9 on gemfibrozil versus 207 on placebo – was comparable. The lack of effect on total mortality was in large part due to a difference in deaths from accidents and violence (10 on gemfibrozil and 3 on placebo).

## ■ MANAGEMENT

Before discussing the merits of available drug treatment strategies, we must confront a crucial but what must ultimately remain an unresolvable issue: whether to assign more weight to improvements in cardiovascular mortality or total mortality.

By pooling all available data from 23 clinical trials involving over 42 000 patients up to the end of 1990, Silberberg found that cholesterol lowering reduced the incidence of both fatal and non-fatal coronary events (20 per cent odds reduction, 95 per cent confidence interval (CI) 14–25 per cent) and coronary mortality (11 per cent odds reduction, 95 per cent CI 3–19 per cent). However, for total mortality the odds reduction was only 2 per cent (95 per cent CI – 5 [excess]-9 per cent)[32] due to a small increase in non-coronary-related deaths.

The medical world is divided into those who believe that a reduction in coronary morbidity is worthwhile and those who believe that only all-cause mortality matters. The excess of non-coronary deaths among those treated with lipid-lowering therapy has been mostly attributable to cancer and trauma (accidents, violence and suicide).

Does this adverse association with lowering serum cholesterol make biological sense? Although some critics have agreed that serum cholesterol concentrations can be linked to mood and that treating hypercholesterolaemia might lead to depression,[33] no convincing clinical evidence exists to support such a hypothesis. Indeed, the different categories of death that are supposedly associated with hypolipidaemic treatment argue against a single causal association. Weak and circumstantial evidence that ties low cholesterol to cancer or violent death and which ignores the potential influences of confounding variables – vitamin A in cancer, for example – should be treated with great caution before rejecting lipid-lowering therapy as either dangerous or lacking efficacy.

How then should a doctor manage a patient with 'hyperlipid-aemia'?

## ☐ Diagnosis

Careful clinical assessment is necessary. This includes noting the age and sex of the patient, their present health, and their past medical history. In addition, a family history must be taken, identifying those who may have had CAD under the age of 65. Finally, other risk factors, especially smoking and diabetes mellitus, should be recorded. Physical examination should include careful inspection for xanthomas, xanthelasmata and early corneal arcus. The cardiovascular system must be carefully examined, with blood pressure, peripheral pulses and the presence or absence of bruits carefully noted.

Common secondary causes of hypercholesterolaemia.

| Fredrickson class | Generic designation | Lipoprotein particle affected |
|---|---|---|
| I | Exogenous hyperlipidaemia | Chylomicrons |
| IIa | Hypercholesterolaemia | LDL |
| IIb | Combined hyperlipidaemia | LDL + VLDL |
| III | Remnant hyperlipidaemia | Remnant particles |
| IV | Endogenous hyperlipidaemia | VLDL |
| V | Mixed hyperlipidaemia | VLDL + chylomicrons |

**Table 3.3** Fredrickson classification of primary hypercholesterolaemias.

There are two important questions to ask. First, is a high serum cholesterol concentration due to a primary or secondary disorder? Secondary causes of hypercholesterolaemia obviously need addressing before any direct intervention to lower serum cholesterol. Second, if the lipid abnormality is primary, what is the key defect? To answer this question, one may adopt either the Fredrickson (Table 3.3) or a genetic (Table 3.4) classification. Measurement of the serum triglyceride concentration is essential to make an accurate diagnosis. Such a detailed assessment is important because of the possible need for family screening.

| Genetic class | Fredrickson type |
|---|---|
| 1. Recessive apolipoprotein disorder | |
| (a) Apoprotein CII deficiency | I, V |
| (b) Familial dysbetalipoproteinaemia | III |
| 2. Dominant receptor mutations | |
| (a) Familial hypercholesterolaemia | IIa |
| 3. Recessive enzyme mutations | |
| (a) Familial lipoprotein lisage deficiency | I, V |
| (b) Familial LCAT deficiency | – |
| 4. Possible monogenic disorders | |
| (a) Familial hypertriglyceridaemia | IV, V |
| (b) Familial multiple-type hyperlipoproteinaemia | IV, IIb |
| 5. Polygenic disorders | |
| (a) Hypercholesterolaemia | IIa |
| (b) Hypertriglyceridaemia | IV |

**Table 3.4** Genetic classification of primary hyperlipoproteinaemias.

# ☐ Initial management

Complex, age-dependent tabulations of risk and management have been proposed by both the National Institutes of Health and the European Atherosclerosis Society.[6] These recommendations have produced enormous controversy and confusion. A simple decision-making strategy is essential for the physician faced with a patient with hypercholesterolaemia.

A normal range for cholesterol is impossible to define but here we provide some simple guidelines.

• A plasma cholesterol concentration of less than 5.2 mmol/l is desirable; anything higher is undesirable. Values over 6.5 mmol/l (about 250 mg/dl) are a cause for concern and those over 7.8 mmol/l (about 300 mg/dl) have about a three-fold increase in risk for coronary events compared with those with a cholesterol of below 5.2 mmol/l. Risk rises sharply for figures above 7.8 mmol/l.

- Coronary risk is influenced by several factors that have an additive adverse effect. Patients who also have other risk factors, which includes being male, merit more vigorous regimens to reduce their cholesterol.
- Patients with a bad family history or who already have clinically evident vascular disease (angina, transient ischaemic attacks, intermittent claudication) merit effective therapy to reduce their total cholesterol below 6 mmol/l.
- Dietary therapy should be tried initially in all patients, drug therapy being introduced early when prognostic indicators suggest the need for more vigorous treatment.

Triglycerides alone probably confer little excess risk of coronary heart disease – unless the patient is diabetic[27] – and do not require specific targeted therapy. However, some recent evidence does point to triglycerides as an independent risk factor for coronary heart disease among men aged over 60 years.[34] Secondary causes of hypertriglyceridaemia should also be ruled out.

In the USA, the National Cholesterol Education Programme recommends a diet containing less than 30 per cent of calories in the form of fat, less than 10 per cent in saturated fat, and less than 300 mg of cholesterol per day.

Browner and colleagues calculated that if all Americans reduced their dietary fat intake to those levels, CAD mortality rates would fall by 5–20 per cent.[35] Overall, about 42 000 of the

Diabetes mellitus
Alcohol
Oral contraceptive pill
Hypothyroidism
Uraemia
Acromegaly

Secondary causes of hypertriglyceridaemia.

2–3 million adult US deaths each year could be prevented. This figure translates into an extended average life expectancy of 3–4 months, which would predominantly benefit those aged over 65 years.

The power of dietary therapy combined with regular exercise in reducing serum cholesterol concentration by up to one-quarter must also be emphasized.[36,37]

## ☐ Drug therapy

There are six main groups of drugs for the treatment of hyperlipidaemias.

- Ion–exchange resins
    Cholestyramine
    Colestipol
- Fibrates
    Bezafibrate
    Gemfibrozil
    Ciprofibrate
    Fenofibrate
- HMG-CoA reductase inhibitors
    Lovastatin
    Pravastatin
    Simvastatin
- Fish oils
    Omega-3 marine triglycerides
- Probucol
- Nicotinic acid derivatives
    Acipimox
    Nicofuranose
    Nicotinic acid

Drug classes for treatment of hyperlipidaemia.

## Ion-exchange resins

Non-absorbable anion-exchange resins, such as cholestyramine and colestipol, act by binding and increasing the faecal excretion of bile salts. More cholesterol is therefore converted into bile acids and LDL cholesterol breakdown is thus accelerated. Large daily doses of cholestyramine (8–24 g) are required and complications include constipation, dyspepsia, flatulence and interference with the absorption of other drugs (e.g. digoxin, thyroxine, and warfarin) and nutrients (iron, folate).

Reduction of LDL cholesterol makes these drugs especially valuable for the treatment of heterozygous FH. Additionally, in the Lipid Research Clinics Primary Prevention Trial,[29] 24 g cholestyramine daily for 7 years led to a mean fall in cholesterol of 8.5 per cent, a mean fall in LDL cholesterol of 12.6 per cent, and a mean increase in HDL cholesterol of 3 per cent compared with those receiving placebo (Figure 3.3). One–third of patients discontinued the drug because of side–effects. Similar findings to these have been reported in the National Heart and Blood Institute's type II coronary intervention study among patients with severe hypercholesterolaemia.[38] Colestipol has a similar mode of action to cholestyramine and is especially valuable in children because of its safety.

This group of drugs has been recommended as first-line therapy for hypercholesterolaemia by the National Cholesterol Education Program.[39]

## Fibrates

Since clofibrate is the only member of this class of drugs to have a clinically important lithogenic effect on bile, its use cannot be recommended.

Gemfibrozil is an effective agent for reducing serum triglycerides. In the Helsinki Heart Study,[30,40] gemfibrozil 600 mg twice daily in over 4000 middle-aged men with a 'primary dyslipidaemia' over a 5-year period reduced total cholesterol by 11 per cent, LDL cholesterol by 10 per cent and triglycerides by 43 per cent (Figure 3.4). HDL cholesterol increased by 10 per cent. The beneficial effects on coronary heart disease – a 35 per cent reduction in cardiac end-points – were due mainly to gemfibrozil's effects on LDL and HDL.

Bezafibrate is an effective agent for reducing both serum cholesterol and triglycerides.[3] For instance, it can reduce serum cholesterol by over 20 per cent in patients with FH.[41]

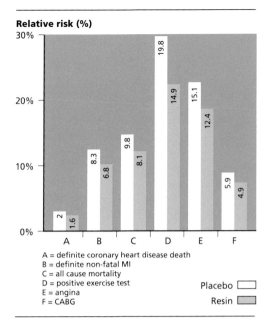

**Relative risk (%)**

A = definite coronary heart disease death
B = definite non-fatal MI
C = all cause mortality
D = positive exercise test
E = angina
F = CABG

Placebo
Resin

**Figure 3.3** Efficacy of cholestyramine resin in modifying cardiovascular events in the Lipid Research Clinics Study. A = definite coronary heart disease death; B = definite non-fatal MI; C = all-cause mortality; D = positive exercise test; E = angina; F = CABG.[29]

Bezafibrate's precise mechanism of action remains unknown, although it may interfere with fatty acid synthesis and peripheral lipolysis.

Newer fibrates (e.g. ciprofibrate, fenofibrate) may have more pronounced effects on LDL cholesterol, but long–term studies are not yet available to confirm such hopes.

### Statins

3-Hydroxy-3-methylglutaryl-CoA is the rate-limiting enzyme in the synthesis of cholesterol. Inhibitors of this enzyme – the

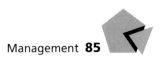

**% Change from baseline**

**Figure 3.4**  Risk reduction of coronary heart disease attributed to alterations in lipid concentrations. A = total cholesterol; B = HDL cholesterol; C = LDL cholesterol; D = triglyceride.[30]

statins – are the most powerful lipid-lowering agents yet produced. A reversible myositis with these agents has been described in about 0.5 per cent of patients, but is rare unless there is concurrent therapy with cyclosporin (in which case, rhabdomyolysis and transient renal failure have been reported), nicotinic acid and gemfibrozil. A mild, transient increase in alanine aminotransferase has also been reported.

Their main action is to lower LDL cholesterol and, in this respect, the statins are more potent than ion-exchange resins. The efficacy of lovastatin has been shown in the EXCEL study (Extended Clinical Evaluation of Lovastatin).[42,43] This randomized,

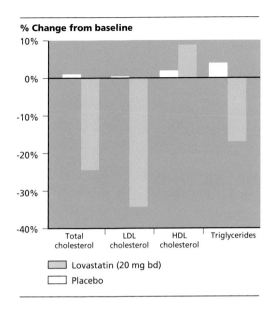

**% Change from baseline**

Lovastatin (20 mg bd)

Placebo

**Figure 3.5**   Changes in lipoprotein profile with lovastatin.[42,43]

double-blind, diet- and placebo-controlled trial among 8245 participants with moderate hypercholesterolaemia (6.21–7.76 mmol/l) found that lovastatin produced dose-dependent reductions in LDL cholesterol ranging from 24 per cent to 40 per cent (Figure 3.5). HDL cholesterol was increased by about 10 per cent, also in a dose-dependent manner. Furthermore, when a low-fat diet was combined with lovastatin, LDL cholesterol fell by 32 per cent.[44] They are less effective than fibrates at reducing serum triglycerides (20 per cent) and in raising HDL cholesterol (5–15 per cent).[45] The benefits of simvastatin therapy are maintained over at least 3 years;[46] longer term experience has not yet been published.

Once-daily pravastatin reduces LDL cholesterol by 20–35 per cent and total cholesterol by 15–25 per cent after 8 weeks of treatment.[47] HDL cholesterol increased by 12 per cent and triglycerides fell by over 20 per cent. Similar changes in lipid profiles were found over a 16-week treatment course.[48] When pravastatin was directly compared with gemfibrozil,[49] the statin produced greater reductions in LDL cholesterol (30 per cent versus 17 per cent), but lower increases in HDL cholesterol (5 per cent versus 13 per cent) and lower falls in triglycerides (5 per cent versus 37 per cent). In direct comparator trials, simvastatin is more potent than both lovastatin[50] and pravastatin[51]

### Nicotinic acid (niacin)

Although nicotinic acid is also a recommended first–line treatment, its use is limited by its side-effect profile. This agent, together with its analogue, acipimox, inhibits VLDL secretion and hence reduces serum cholesterol concentrations. Adverse effects include liver damage, which occurs even with low-dose, short-term therapy,[52] gastrointestinal symptoms and flushing. Nicotinic acid may also be arrhythmogenic.

The Coronary Drug Project[31] showed reductions in cholesterol and triglycerides of 10 per cent and 28 per cent, respectively (Figure 3.6) . HDL concentration was also reduced. Nicotinic acid seems to reduce both coronary *and* total mortality. Benefits of treatment with this vitamin were also seen in the CLAS[53] and FATS[54] protocols.

### Probucol

This anti–oxidant reduces serum LDL cholesterol concentrations by 10–20 per cent.[55,56] It has little effect on serum triglycerides. Of particular interest is the finding that probucol substantially reduces measures of lipid peroxidation in hypercholesterolaemic patients.[57] This observation raises the possibility that probucol will become a valuable co-therapy with other more powerful lipid-lowering agents.[58]

### Fish oils

Fish oils are rich in omega-3 fatty acids (eicosapentanoic acid, eicosahexanoic acid and docosahexanoic acid). Reductions are achieved in VLDL cholesterol, especially triglycerides. For example, when 20–30 per cent of calories are provided by fish oil derivatives, cholesterol and triglyceride concentrations can be substantially diminished.[59] There is also concern that fish oils can

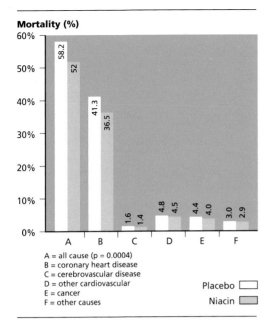

**Figure 3.6** Coronary Drug Project mortality by cause for a mean follow-up period of 15 years. A = all cause ($p$ = 0.0004); B = coronary heart disease; C = cerebrovascular disease; D = other cardiovascular; E = cancer; F = other causes.[31]

increase circulating LDL cholesterol concentrations in some circumstances (type IV hyperlipidaemia, for example).[60]

The main role of this drug class is for treating hypertriglyceridaemia, but the high doses that are necessary limit compliance.

## ☐ Radical measures to treat hyperlipidaemia

In patients with severe FH or in those in whom drug therapy fails, more radical interventions may be necessary.

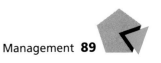

Plasma exchange at 2-weekly intervals involves exchanging 2–4 l plasma for plasma protein fraction. Co-therapy with drugs, such as the statins, may also be beneficial.[61] LDL apheresis (selective removal of VLDL and LDL by affinity chromatography) can reduce serum cholesterol by up to 50 per cent but must also be done every 2 weeks.[62,63] Apheresis is the treatment of choice for homozygous FH.

Surgical intervention with partial ileal bypass (to diminish bile salt reabsorption)[64] or even liver transplantation[65] can also be successful in selected cases.

Gene therapy, in which genes coding for defective receptors or enzymes (Table 3.4), may also prove valuable in the future. Transgenic animal models confirm the practicability of such an approach.[66]

# ■ CONCLUSION

## □ Management guidelines

We have seen that, with a long enough follow-up, it is likely that benefits not only in cardiovascular mortality but also in total mortality will be seen with lipid-lowering therapy.[39]

Therapeutic decisions are, on the basis of the limited data so far available, clearly difficult to make with certainty. However, once a decision to treat has been made, we recommend the following protocol:

---

- **High total cholesterol:**
    Single agent – resin *or* fibrate *or* statin
    Combination – resin + statin

- **High triglyceride:**
    Single agent – gemfibrozil
    Combination – add nicotinic acid

---

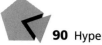

Three outstanding questions remain.

1. How does the prescriber judge when to initiate treatment?
2. Does measurement of LDL confer any additional benefit to that of total cholesterol?
3. How important is a high triglyceride and/or a low HDL concentration?

## ☐ When to treat

Points in the patient's history should act as triggers to adopt a more aggressive approach – earlier drug therapy – when combined with an assessment of total cholesterol. These triggers include:

• Smoking history
• Family history of coronary heart disease
• Hypertension[67]
• Diabetes
• High waist/hip ratio (male fat distribution)[68]

Moreover, treatment with lipid-lowering agents should be combined not only with traditional risk factor intervention (modification of the above variables) but also with exercise programmes. Exercise is cardioprotective in its own right and is an important non-pharmacological part of treating the patient at cardiac risk.[69]

Finally, evidence of benefit from treatment exists in the setting of both primary prevention[35,48,49] and, although more contentiously, secondary prevention.[39,70]

## ☐ Measurement of LDL

One-third of MIs take place with total cholesterol (TC) concentrations below 5.2 mmol/l – i.e. within that range normally classified as 'desirable'. LDL is a far more accurate measure for judging risk but the multiplicity of formulas for assessing the influence of LDL has led only to confusion. For example, one can select the Friedewald equation,

$$LDL = TC - HDL + \frac{TG}{5}$$

or the cholesterol retention fraction,

$$CRF = \frac{LDL - HDL}{LDL}$$

or the Framingham fraction,

$$FF = \frac{TC}{HDL}$$

This confusion will soon be resolved by the introduction in the USA of a Food and Drug Administration approved LDL assay made by Genzyme. Assessment of broad risk categories will then become much easier (Table 3.5).

| | Desirable | Borderline | Abnormal |
|---|---|---|---|
| Total cholesterol | <5.2 | 5.2–6.2 | >6.2 |
| LDL cholesterol | <4.0 | 4.0–5.0 | >5.0 |
| HDL cholesterol | >1.0 | 0.9–1.0 | >0.9 |
| Triglyceride | <2.0 | 2.0–2.5 | >2.5 |

**Table 3.5** Decision-making categories in lipid evaluation.

## ☐ High triglyceride, low HDL

Although many observers intuitively believe that these variables are important, there are no clear prospective data to prove that intervention to modify these lipid fractions produces any benefit.[71] However, since 50 per cent of MIs occur in people with LDL concentrations below 4.0 mmol/l, HDL and triglycerides are likely to influence risk significantly.

In a patient with a normal total cholesterol and a normal LDL, but who has a trigger factor, we would recommend treatment of high serum triglycerides (as described above). We realize that few data exist to support such an assertion, but since a large proportion of cardiac events take place when cholesterol/LDL concentrations are normal, to leave a high triglyceride untreated, together with (an)other trigger factor(s), is likely to be a high-risk non-intervention strategy.

HDL concentrations are inversely correlated with triglyceride concentrations and it is quite common to find low HDL with high triglyceride. This combination is high risk.[72] Intervention in such cases reduces this risk.[49] We believe that a fibrate or nicotinic acid is indicated in these cases.

An isolated low HDL does not require specific treatment unless additional trigger factors are present. However, it would not be unreasonable for clinicians who face patients with low HDL concentrations plus several trigger factors to begin treatment to correct the HDL abnormality.

## References

**1.** Kern F, Normal plasma cholesterol in an 88-year-old man who eats 25 eggs a day: mechanisms of adaptation, *N Engl J Med* (1991) **324**:896–99.

**2.** Skrabanek P, The diet/heart crusade In: Mann GV, ed., *Coronary heart disease: the dietary sense and nonsense*, (Janus: London 1993) 94–102.

**3.** Henkin Y, Kreisberg RA, Progression, stabilization, and regression of coronary heart disease: effects of lipoprotein modification. In: Kreisberg RA, Segrest JP, eds, *Plasma lipoprotein and coronary artery disease*, (Blackwell: Oxford 1992) 29–54.

**4.** Fredrickson DS, Levy RI, Lees RS, Fat transport in lipoproteins: an integrated approach to mechanisms and disorders, *N Engl J Med* (1967) **276**:34–44, 94–103, 148–56, 215–23, 273–81.

**5.** Gotto AM, Pownall HJ, Havell RJ, Introduction to the plasma lipoproteins. *Methods enzymol* (1986) 3–41.

**6.** McIntyre N, Harry DS, *Lipids and lipoproteins in clinical practice* (Wolfe: London, 1991).

**7.** Goldstein JL, Brown MS, Regulation of low density lipoprotein receptors: implications for pathogenesis and therapy of hypercholesterolaemia and atherosclerosis, *Circulation* (1987) **76**:504–7.

**8.** Ross R, Harker L, Hyperlipidaemia and atherosclerosis, *Science* (1976) **193**:1094–100.

**9.** Ross R, The pathogenesis of atherosclerosis – an update, *N Engl J Med* (1986) **314**:488–500.

**10.** Aqed NM, Ball RY, Waldmann H, Mitchinson MH, Monocytic origin of foam cells in human atherosclerotic plaques, *Atherosclerosis* (1984) **53**:265–71.

**11.** Steinbrecher UP, Zhang H, Loughead M, Role of oxidatively modified LDL in atherosclerosis, *Free Radic Biol Med* (1990) **9**:155–68.

**12.** Steinberg D, Parthasarathy S, Carew TE, Khoo JC, Witztum JL, Beyond cholesterol: modifications of low-density lipoproteins that increase its atherogenicity, *N Engl J Med* (1989) **320**:915–23.

**13.** McGill HC, McMahan CA, Kruski AW, Mott GE, Relationship of lipoprotein cholesterol concentrations to experimental atherosclerosis in baboons, *Arteriosclerosis* (1981) **1**:3–12.

**14.** Levy RI, Brensike JF, Epstein SE et al, The influence of changes in lipid values induced by cholestyramine and diet on progression of coronary artery disease: results of the NHLDI type II coronary intervention study, *Circulation* (1984) **69**:325–37.

**15.** Blankenhorn DH, Wessim SA, Johnson RL et al, Beneficial effects of combined colestipol–niacin therapy on coronary atherosclerosis and coronary venous bypass grafts, *JAMA* (1987) **257**:3233–40.

**16.** Keys A, Coronary heart disease in seven countries, *Circulation* (1970) **41**:1–21.

**17.** Mann GV (ed.), *Coronary heart disease: the dietary sense and nonsense* (Janus: London, 1993).

**18.** Goldstein JL, Hazzard WE, Schrott HG, Bierman EL, Motulsky AG, Hyperlipidaemia in coronary heart disease: I, lipid levels in 500 survivors of myocardial infarction, *J Clin Invest* (1973) **52**:1533–43.

**19.** Kannel WB, Dawber TR, Kagan A, Devotskie N, Stokes J, Factors of risk in the development of coronary heart disease: six year follow-up experience (the Framingham Study), *Ann Intern Med* (1961) **55**:33–50.

**20.** Martin MJ, Hulley SB, Browner WS, Kuller LH, Wentworth D, Serum cholesterol, blood pressure and mortality: implications from a cohort of 361662 men, *Lancet* (1986) **ii**:933–6.

**21.** Barbir M, Wile D, Trayner I, Aber VR, Thompson GR, High prevalence of hyper-triglyceridaemia and apolipoprotein abnor-malities in coronary artery disease, *Br Heart J* (1988) **60**:397–403.

**22.** Castelli WP, Garrison RJ, Wilson PWF et al, Incidence of coronary heart disease and lipoprotein cholesterol levels, *JAMA* (1986) **256**:2835–8.

**23.** Romm PA, Green CE, Reagan K, Rackley CE, Relation of serum lipoprotein cholesterol levels to presence and severity of angiographic coronary artery disease, *Am J Cardiol* (1991) **67**:479–83.

**24.** Hong MK, Romm PA, Reagan K, Green CE, Rackley CE, Usefulness of the total cholesterol to HDL cholesterol ratio in predicting angiographic coronary artery disease in women, *Am J Cardiol* (1991) **68**:1646–50.

**25.** Salonen JT, Salonen R, Seppanen K, Rauramaar, Tuomilehto J, HDL, $HDL_2$, and HDL$_3$ subfractions and the risk of acute myocardial infarction: a prospective popula-tion study in eastern Finnish men, *Circulation* (1991) **84**:129–39.

**26.** Stampfer MJ, Sacks FM, Salvini S, Willett WC, Hennekens CH, A prospective study of cholesterol, apolipoproteins, and the risk of myocardial infarction, *N Engl J Med* (1991) **325**:373–81.

**27.** Criqui MH, Heiss G, Cohn R et al, Plasma triglyceride level and mortality from coronary heart disease, *N Engl J Med* (1993) **328**:1220–5.

**28.** Lobo KA, Notelovitz M, Bernstein L et al, Lp(a) lipoprotein: relationship to cardio-vascular disease risk factors, exercise, and estrogen, *Am J Obstet Gynecol* (1992) **166**:1182–90.

**29.** Lipid Research Clinics Program, The Lipid Research Clinics Coronary Primary Prevention Trial results.1. Reductions in incidence of coronary heart disease, *JAMA* (1984) **251**:351–64.

**30.** Frick MH, Elo O, Haapa et al, Helsinki Heart Study: primary prevention trial with gemfibrozil in middle–aged men with dyslipid-aemia, *N Engl J Med* (1987) **317**:1237–45.

**31.** Canner PL, Berge KG, Wenger NK et al, Fifteen year mortality in coronary drug project patients: long-term benefit with niacin, *J Am Coll Cardiol* (1986) **8**:1245–55.

**32.** Silberberg JS, Meta-analysis of clinical trials of lipid-lowering therapies. Consensus conference on hyperlipidaemia, Canberra, Australia, 1991. [abstr.]

**33.** Engleberg H, Low serum cholesterol and suicide, *Lancet* (1992) **339**:727–9.

**34.** Welin L, Eriksson H, Ohlson LO et al, Triglycerides, a major coronary risk factor in elderly men: a study of men born in 1913, *Eur Heart J* (1991) **12**:700–4.

**35.** Browner WS, Westenhouse J, Tice JA, What if Americans ate less fat? A quantita-tive effect of the effect on mortality, *JAMA* (1991) **265**:3285–91.

**36.** Barnard RJ, Effects of life-style modifica-tion on serum lipids, *Arch Intern Med* (1991) **151**:1389–94.

**37.** Wood PD, Stefanick ML, Williams PT, Haskell WL, The effects on plasma lipopro-teins of a prudent weight reducing diet, with or without exercise, in overweight men and women, *N Engl J Med* (1991) **325**:461–6.

**38.** Levy RI, Brensicke JF, Epstein SE et al, The influences of changes in lipid values induced by cholestyramine and diet on progression of coronary artery disease: results of the NHLBI type II coronary intervention study, *Circulation* (1984) **69**:325–37.

**39.** The Expert Panel. Report of the National Cholesterol Education Program Expert Panel on detection, evaluation, and treatment of high blood cholesterol in adults, *Arch Intern Med* (1988) **148**:36–69.

**40.** Manninen V, Elo O, Frick MH, Lipid alterations and decline in the incidence of coronary heart disease in the Helsinki Heart Study, *JAMA* (1988) **260**:641–51.

**41.** Wheeler KAH, West RJ, Lloyd JK, Barley J, Double-blind trial of bezafibrate in familial hypercholesterolaemia, *Arch Dis Child* (1985) **60**:34–7.

**42.** Bradford RH, Shear CL, Chremos AN et al, Expanded clinical Evaluation of Lovastatin (EXCEL) Study Results, *Arch Intern Med* (1991) **151**:43–9.

**43.** Shear CL, Cranklin FA, Stinnett S et al, Expanded Clinical Evaluation of Lovastatin (EXCEL) Study Results, *Circulation* (1992) **85**:1293–303.

**44.** Hunninghake DB, Stein EA, Dujorne CA et al, The efficacy of intensive dietary therapy alone or combined with lovastatin in outpatients with hypercholesterolaemia, *N Engl J Med* (1993) **328**:1213–19.

**45.** Hoogerbrugge An D, Mol MTN, Van Dormaal JJ et al, The efficacy and safety of pravastatin compared to and in combination with bile acid binding resins in familial hypercholesterolaemia, *J Intern Med* (1990) **228**:261–6.

**46.** Boccuzzi SJ, Bocanegra TS, Walker JF, Shapiro DR, Keegan ME, Long-term safety and efficacy profile of simvastatin, *Am J Cardiol* (1991) **68**:1127–31.

**47.** Jones PH, Farmer JA, Cressman MD et al, Once daily pravastatin in patients with primary hypercholesterolaemia: a dose response study, *Clin Cardiol* (1991) **14**:146–51.

**48.** Rubenfire M, Maciejko JJ, Blevins RD et al, The effect of pravastatin on plasma

lipoprotein and apolipoprotein levels in primary hypercholesterolaemia, *Arch Intern Med* (1991) **151**:2234–40.

**49.** Cvepaldi G, Baggio G, Area M et al, Pravastatin vs gemfibrozil in the treatment of primary hypercholesterolaemia: the Italian multicentre pravastatin study, *Arch Intern Med* (1991) **151**:146–52.

**50.** Farmer JA, Washington LC, Jones PH et al, Comparative effects of simvastatin and lovastatin in patients with hypercholesterolaemia, *Clin Ther* (1992) **14**:708–17.

**51.** European Study Group, Efficacy and tolerability of simvastatin and pravastatin in patients with primary hypercholesterolaemia, *Am J Cardiol* (1992) **70**:1281–6.

**52.** Etchason JA, Miller TD, Squires RW et al, Niacin-induced hepatitis: a potential side-effect with low-dose time-release niacin, *Mayo Clin Proc* (1991) **66**:23–8.

**53.** Blankenhorn DH, Nessim SA, Johnson RL et al, Beneficial effects of combined colestipol–niacin therapy on coronary atherosclerosis and coronary venous bypass grafts, *JAMA* (1987) **257**:3233–40.

**54.** Brown G, Albers JJ, Fisher LD et al, Regression of coronary artery disease as a result of intensive lipid-lowering therapy in men with high levels of apolipoprotein B, *N Engl J Med* (1990) **323**:1289–98.

**55.** Buckley MMT, Goa KL, Price AH, Brogden RN, Probucol: a reappraisal of its pharmacological properties and therapeutic use in hypercholesterolaemia, *Drugs* (1989) **37**:761–800.

**56.** Witztum JL, Simmons D, Steinberg D et al, Intensive combination drug therapy of familial hypercholesterolaemia with lovastatin, probucol, and colestipol hydrochloride, *Circulation* (1989) **79**:16–28.

**57.** Masana L, Bargallo T, Plana N et al, Effectiveness of probucol in inducing plasma low-density lipoprotein cholesterol oxidation in hypercholesterolaemia, *Am J Cardiol* (1991) **68**:863–7.

**58.** Steinberg D, Parthasarathy S, Carew TE, Khoo JC, Witztum JL, Beyond cholesterol: modifications of low-density lipoprotein that increase its atherogenicity, *N Engl J Med* (1989) **320**:915–24.

**59.** Phillipson BE, Rothbock DW, Connor WE, Harris WS, Illingworth DR, Reduction of plasma lipids, lipoproteins, and apoproteins of dietary fish oils in patients with hypertriglyceridaemia, *N Engl J Med* (1985) **312**:1210–16.

**60.** Thompson GR: Lipids, fish, and coronary heart disease, *Curr Opin Cardiol* (1986) **1**:827–31.

**61.** Thompson GR, Ford J, Jenkinson M, Trayner I, Efficacy of mevinolin as adjuvant therapy for refractory familial hypercholesterolaemia, *Q J Med* (1986) **60**:803–11.

**62.** Yokoyama S, Haashi R, Satani M, Yamamoto A, Selective removal of low density lipoprotein by plasmapheresis in familial hypercholesterolaemia, *Arteriosclerosis* (1985) **5**:613–22.

**63.** Mabuchi H, Michishita I, Takeda M et al, A new LDL apheresis system using two dextran sulphate cellulose columns in an automated column regenerating unit, *Atherosclerosis* (1987) **68**:19–26.

**64.** Buchwald H, Varzo RL, Matts JP et al, The effect of partial ileal bypass surgery on mortality and morbidity from coronary heart disease in patients with hypercholesterolaemia, *N Engl J Med*(1990) **323**:946–55.

**65.** Starzl TE, Bilheimer DW, Bahnson HT et al, Heart–liver transplantation in a patient with familial hypercholesterolaemia, *Lancet* (1984) **i**:1382–3.

**66.** Hoffmann SL, Russell DW, Brown MS, Goldstein JL, Hammer RE, Overexpression of LDL receptor eliminates LDL from plasma in transgenic mice, *Science* (1988) **239**:1277–81.

**67.** Bonna KH, Thelle DS, Association between blood pressure and serum lipids in a population – The Tromso study, *Circulation* (1991) **83**:1305–14.

**68.** Thompson CJ, Ryu JE, Craven TE, Kahl FR, Crovse JR, Central adipose distribution is related to coronary atherosclerosis, *Arterioscl Thromb* (1991) **II**:327–33.

**69.** Ornish D, Brown SE, Schermitz LW et al, Can lifestyle changes reverse coronary heart disease: the Lifestyle Heart Trial, *Lancet* (1990) **336**:129–33.

**70.** Carlson LA, Rosenhamer G, Reduction of mortality in the Stockholm Ischaemic Heart Disease Secondary Prevention Study by combined treatment with clofibrate and nicotinic acid, *Acta Med Scand* (1988) **223**:405–18.

**71.** NIH Consensus Development Panel on Triglyceride, High-Density Lipoprotein, and Coronary Heart Disease, Triglyceride, high-density lipoprotein, and coronary heart disease, *JAMA* (1993) **269**:505–10.

**72.** Castelli WP, The triglyceride issue: a view from Framingham, *Am Heart J* (1986) **112**:432–7.

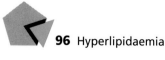

# Chapter 4
# **Thromboembolism**

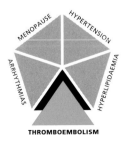

In many ways, the issue of thromboembolism provides the simplest treatment decisions for the clinician who is attempting to prevent coronary events. We will consider the therapeutic efficacy of antithrombotic therapy in the format shown in Table 4.1.

There is, of course, a vascular phase that precedes the platelet – that is, endothelial injury (plaque formation or hypertension) leads to exposure of a subendothelial vascular wall matrix, together with release of ADP and tissue thromboplastin. These events are dealt with elsewhere under lipid-lowering therapy and antihypertensive treatment.

Furthermore, our focus is the long-term cardioprotective management of the patient at risk of coronary disease. Acute management with thrombolytics, aspirin and heparin is not our primary concern, although we must briefly review the current position of these treatments to place what follows in the wider context of thromboembolic risk.

First, however, we will give a brief but essential summary of the physiology of human haemostatic mechanisms.

| Haemostatic phase | Primary prevention | Secondary prevention |
| --- | --- | --- |
| Platelet phase | Aspirin | Aspirin |
| Coagulation phase | | Heparin, warfarin |
| Fibrinolytic phase | | Thrombolytics |

**Table 4.I** Antithrombotic treatment strategies.

## ■ PHYSIOLOGY OF HAEMOSTASIS

Endothelial cells play a central part in preventing vascular thrombosis. However, once endothelial integrity has been breached, there follows a cascade of events – release of ADP (a platelet aggregation factor) and tissue thromboplastin (tissue

> - Preservation of a transmural negative electrical potential, thereby preventing adhesion of circulating platelets
> - Release of antiplatelet agents, e.g. prostacyclin (PGI$_2$)
> - Release of anticoagulants, e.g. protein C activation (plus thrombomodulin), heparin-like proteoglycans
> - Release of fibrinolytics, e.g. plasminogen activators

Endothelial mechanisms of antithrombosis.

factor, a lipoprotein peptidase) – which leads to platelet activation by binding to factor VIII/vWF polymers and fibronectin, themselves released into the subendothelial matrix by endothelial cells. Platelet shape changes take place, the platelet adheres to the tissue matrix, and a release reaction ensues. Further ADP is secreted from platelet granules and a platelet phospholipase A$_2$ is activated. Thromboxane A$_2$ is subsequently generated, which leads to platelet aggregation. The further recruitment of platelets to the growing thrombus amplifies the release reaction.

Several other factors are produced during the release reaction, all of which will adversely effect the outcome of the patient at coronary risk:

- Serotonin – may cause coronary vasospasm.
- Platelet factor 4 – neutralizes the anticoagulant actions of circulating heparin.
- Platelet-derived growth factor – enhances smooth muscle cell proliferation and promotes atherogenesis.
- Platelet factor 3 – activates several circulating clotting factors.

Coagulation systems are divided into intrinsic and extrinsic. Their linked protease reactions convert proenzymes (inactive coagulation factors) into active enzymes.

The intrinsic system is activated after extravasation (in vitro, by contact with glass, kaolin and phospholipid), a process that involves factors XI and XII and a kininogen–prekallikrein complex. The extrinsic system relies on activation of factor VII

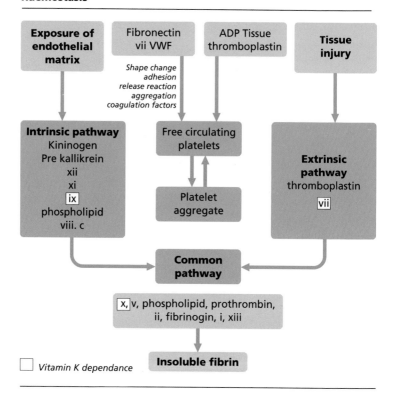

**Figure 4.1** Haemostasis. Bold factors indicate vitamin K dependence. Modified from Wintrobe MM et al, *Clinical Haematology*, 7th edn (Lea and Febiger: Philadelphia 1974) 390, 422.

to VIIa by tissue thromboplastin. These processes are summarized in Figure 4.1.

The fibrinolytic system limits thrombus formation and promotes clot lysis as the wound heals. Figure 4.2 shows the key steps. Plasminogen is converted to plasmin, a protease not normally found in the blood. Plasmin breaks fibrin down into fibrin degradation products. Plasmin generation is initiated by

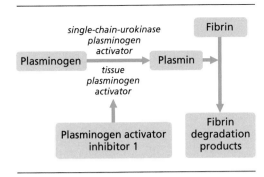

**Figure 4.2** The fibrinolytic system.

two plasminogen activators: tissue plasminogen activator (tPA) and single-chain urokinase plasminogen activator (scu-PA). tPA is inhibited in plasma by plasminogen activator inhibitors (PAI-1 or PAI-2), which are also derived from the endothelium. tPA and scu-PA bind selectively to fibrin on the thrombus surface. Plasminogen binds to this complex and is then converted to plasmin; hence the therapeutic thrombus specificity of the plasminogen activators. Alpha$_2$-antiplasmin is a natural inhibitor of plasmin.

# ■ ACUTE MANAGEMENT

Thrombolytic therapy given within 12 h of onset of symptoms reduces mortality by about 25 per cent, irrespective of age, sex, blood pressure, and site of myocardial infarction (MI) (anterior or inferior) (Fibrinolytic Therapy Trialists' Collaboration, unpublished observations in over 58 000 patients randomized in clinical trials). Aspirin 160 mg on admission and daily thereafter has an additive effect in reducing mortality and should be given to all patients as early as possible.

The debate has moved from *whether* thrombolysis works to *which* agent is most effective. The 'gridlock' in thrombolytic therapy – for example, ISIS-3[1] and GISSI-2[2] showed no difference in efficacy between tPA and streptokinase – seems to have been broken by the GUSTO (Global Utilisation of Streptokinase and tPA for Occluded Coronary Arteries) trial results.[3]

GUSTO enrolled 41 021 patients with an acute MI from over 1000 centres in 16 countries. Patients were randomized to receive one of four treatment regimens:

- Accelerated tPA (given over 90 min rather than the currently recommended 3 h) + intravenous heparin
- tPA (usual regimen) + streptokinase + intravenous heparin
- Streptokinase + subcutaneous heparin
- Streptokinase + intravenous heparin

The accelerated tPA regimen reduced deaths from MI by 14 per cent compared with the tPA/streptokinase/intravenous heparin group, but was also associated with a higher risk of in-hospital stroke (1–2 per 1000; Table 4.2). Additionally, the efficacy of intravenous heparin when combined with tPA is now settled by

| Treatment regimen | Mortality (%) | Disabling stroke (%) |
|---|---|---|
| Accelerated tPA + i.v. heparin | 6.3 | 0.6 |
| tPA + SK + i.v. heparin | 7.0 | 0.6 |
| SK + s.c. heparin | 7.2 | 0.5 |
| SK + i.v. heparin | 7.4 | 0.5 |

tPA = tissue plasminogen activator
SK = streptokinase

**Table 4.2** GUSTO: 30-day mortality and stroke rates.

GUSTO. The potential cost implications of this result have yet to be addressed.

Some observers claim that a meta-analysis of all thrombolytic agents will put GUSTO into its proper context, and thus may eliminate the advantage of tPA. But the accelerated-dose regimen precludes combination of GUSTO with existing tPA data. Yet the question of acute treatment has now moved beyond even thrombolysis. A series of recent papers has suggested a superior cardioprotective efficacy of immediate percutaneous transluminal coronary angioplasty over both tPA[4] and strepto-kinase.[5] The ISIS-4 trial will examine whether there is any added benefit from nitrate or magnesium therapy above that of streptokinase. The proven efficacy of heparin with tPA will also provide added impetus to research into anticoagulants that are easier to administer and control, e.g. platelet activation inhibitors,[6] thrombin inhibitors, such as the recombinant hirudins,[7] and antibodies against the platelet receptor of adhesive proteins (glycoprotein IIb/IIIa).

# ■ CHRONIC MANAGEMENT

## □ Primary prevention

In patients without a history of vascular disease, there is no conclusive benefit of treatment with antiplatelet agents.[8] The UK trial in British physicians[9] enrolled 5139 healthy male doctors over a 10-year period and openly randomized them to 500 mg aspirin/day (or 330 mg enteric-coated aspirin) or to a control group. Although there was a 15 per cent reduction in mortality in the treated group, this did not achieve statistical significance (Figure 4.3). Moreover, no difference was found for non-fatal MI or stroke. Of most concern was a small excess of strokes in the treatment group.

The report of the US Physicians' Health Study[10] indicated that aspirin (325 mg aspirin on alternate days versus placebo in over 22 000 subjects aged 40–84 years) reduced the rate of both fatal and non-fatal MI, although the total number of cardiovascular deaths in both treatment and control groups was the same (an

**Per 10,000 man years**

**Figure 4.3**
The UK physicians study.

Control

Asprin

* = 2P < 0.05

excess of stroke and sudden death in the aspirin group) (Figure 4.4). This adverse 'trade–off' argues against primary prevention with aspirin. The US study also has serious drawbacks. The data and safety monitoring board stopped the trial at the halfway point and so further information on adverse events is limited. Moreover, extrapolation from a group of physicians to the general population could be regarded as optimistic or pessimistic, depending on your point of view.[11]

In patients with unstable angina, aspirin (75 mg/day) will reduce the risk of an MI and death by about one-third.[12] This result substantiates data from three previous studies (Table 4.3).[13–15] Moreover, in patients with unstable angina refractory to triple therapy with a nitrate, a calcium antagonist and a beta-blocker, an intravenous heparin infusion significantly reduces the frequency of angina, episodes of silent ischaemia and total duration of ischaemia.[16]

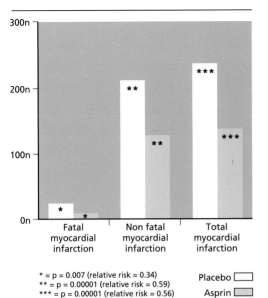

**Figure 4.4**
US physicians health study. MI = myocardial infarction; RR = relative risk. *p = 0.007 (RR = 0.34); **p < 0.00001 (RR = 0.59); ***p < 0.00001 (RR = 0.56).

* = p = 0.007 (relative risk = 0.34)
** = p = 0.00001 (relative risk = 0.59)
*** = p = 0.00001 (relative risk = 0.56)

Placebo ☐
Asprin ☐

| Trial | n | Aspirin dose | End-points that reached statistical significance in favour of aspirin |
|---|---|---|---|
| VA (1983)[13] | 1266 | 324 mg/day | Combined MI + death; non-fatal MI |
| Canadian (1985)[14] | 279 | 1.3 g/day | Cardiac death; total deaths |
| Montreal (1988)[15] | 239 | 650 mg/day | MI |
| RISC (1990)[12] | 796 | 75 mg/day | Combined MI + death |

MI = myocardial infarction

**Table 4.3** Aspirin in unstable angina.

## ☐ Secondary prevention

### Antiplatelet agents

By 1980, six trials had investigated aspirin as a secondary preventive agent. A pooled analysis of these data[17] suggested that there was a clear benefit – a 10 per cent reduction in mortality and a 21 per cent reduction in reinfarction rate – for patients taking 1 g aspirin per day. The PARIS I[18] and PARIS II[19] studies confirmed this fall in reinfarction rate with this dose of aspirin.

In 1988, the Antiplatelet Trialists' Collaboration reported an analysis of 31 randomized trials on the role of aspirin in the prevention of both fatal and non-fatal MI and stroke in survivors of MI or in subjects with unstable angina or who had had transient ischaemic attacks or ischaemic strokes.[20] The main finding for secondary prevention of MI was a reduction of one-quarter in serious vascular events (14 per cent on aspirin versus 18 per cent in control groups) among 18 000 patients from 10 trials.

This meta-analysis was given added weight by the results of the ISIS-2 trial.[21] This study enrolled over 17 000 patients who were randomized to streptokinase and/or aspirin; aspirin (160 mg/day enteric coated) was given for 4 weeks. Aspirin alone produced a 25 per cent odds reduction in vascular mortality, which when given with streptokinase, increased to a 42 per cent fall in the same odds ratio (Table 4.4). ISIS-2 shows that aspirin 160 mg/day for 1 month would avoid 25 deaths and 10–15 reinfarctions and strokes per 1000 treated patients. One can add a further saving of 20 deaths over the subsequent 2–3 years with continuation of aspirin treatment if the results of the Antiplatelet Trialists' Collaboration are also taken into account.

### Oral anticoagulants

The in-hospital mortality of patients following an acute MI, even with modern thrombolysis, is about 10 per cent. A further 10 per cent of patients die within 1 year of hospital discharge, beyond which mortality rates level out at 1–3 per cent per year. How might this high-risk 20 per cent be better managed? Might oral anticoagulants have a role?

The question of oral anticoagulant efficacy post-thrombolytic therapy has not been addressed in a clinical trial. However, an encouraging finding from one of the thrombolysis trials does suggest that this group of drugs should receive further attention.

| | Streptokinase | No streptokinase | Aspirin | No aspirin | Streptokinase and aspirin | Neither |
|---|---|---|---|---|---|---|
| Vascular mortality | 791 | 1029 | 804 | 1016 | 343 | 568 |
| Non-fatal MI | 238 | 202 | 156 | 284 | 77 | 123 |
| Non-fatal stroke | 37 | 41 | 27 | 51 | 13 | 27 |
| Cerebral haemorrhage | 7 | 0 | 5 | 2 | 5 | 0 |

**Table 4.4** The ISIS-II study.

In the AIMS trial,[22] after treatment with anistreplase or placebo plus heparin, warfarin was substituted for heparin and was continued for over 3 months in both groups. The in-hospital reduction in mortality (50.5 per cent) in the group receiving thrombolysis plus warfarin was the highest found in any thrombolytic trial.

A retrospective analysis of 129 patients who had received thrombolytic therapy also indicated a potential benefit from oral anticoagulation.[23] For those receiving warfarin, the rate of cumulative recurrent cardiac events (e.g. unstable angina and reinfarction) at 30 months was 16 per cent in the warfarin group and 39 per cent in a group receiving aspirin: a reduction of almost 60 per cent.

In the Sixty Plus Trial,[24] patients aged over 60 years (mean 67.6) who were receiving oral anticoagulants for at least 6 months after their index cardiac event were randomized to cessation or continuation of treatment. Mortality was reduced by 26 per cent and reinfarction rate fell by 55 per cent in the group continuing anticoagulant therapy. The frequency of intracranial haemorrhage was 1.6 per cent.

The Warfarin Reinfarction Study[25] compared warfarin and placebo for 37 months in 1214 patients (mean age 61.5 years), a mean of 27 days post MI. On warfarin, total mortality fell by 24 per cent, reinfarction rate fell by 34 per cent and stroke rates fell by 55 per cent. The frequency of intracranial haemorrhage was 0.8 per cent: thus, when compared with the Sixty Plus trial, risk seems related to age.

These beneficial effects of oral anticoagulants are rarely discussed.

# ■ CONCLUSION

One can summarize the importance of treating (potential) thromboembolism associated with coronary artery disease (Figure 4.5) as follows:

- Aspirin reduces deaths from myocardial infarction in patients with unstable coronary artery disease (CAD) by one-third, but is of no proven benefit in those without a history of vascular disease.

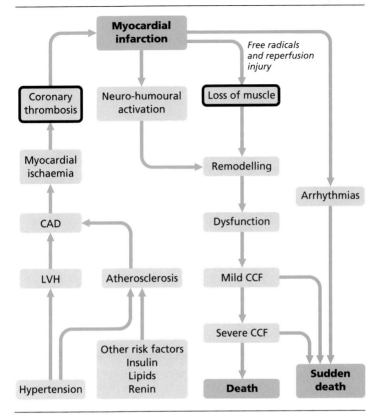

**Figure 4.5**  Interventions to limit thromboembolism in the ischaemic cycle.

- Secondary prevention with aspirin both in the short and long term saves about 45 deaths per 1000 patients treated.
- Oral anticoagulants probably reduce mortality post-MI by about one-quarter, although this estimate requires formal confirmation in a randomized, controlled trial.

What of the future? The indications for antiplatelet therapy may be extended further. For example, in men with chronic stable angina, 325 mg aspirin on alternate days seems to produce an 86 per cent risk reduction for subsequent rates of MI.[26] This result was derived from a subgroup analysis of the US Physicians' Health Study and requires replication in a large clinical trial. The benefits of primary prevention with aspirin in women might also be a surprise finding when tested prospectively.[27]

Low-dose oral anticoagulation is currently under investigation in the Thrombosis Prevention Trial.[28] In this study, men at risk of coronary heart disease but who have not yet had an MI are being randomized to receive low-intensity oral anticoagulation with warfarin (INR 1.5) plus or minus aspirin.

Finally, prethrombotic states may predispose those who have cardiovascular risk factors to an increased frequency of coronary events.[29] If such individuals can be identified – e.g. those with abnormal platelet function tests, high concentrations of PAI-1, protein C or protein S abnormalities, and other molecular markers of a predisposition to thrombosis – then targeted prophylaxis may be more effective than a global population-based approach.

### References

**1.** ISIS-3 (Third International Study of Infarct Survival) Collaborative Group, A randomised comparison of streptokinase vs tissue plasminogen activator vs antistreplase and of aspirin plus heparin vs aspirin alone among 41 299 cases of suspected acute myocardial infarction, *Lancet* (1992) **339**:753–70.

**2.** The International Study Group, In-hospital mortality and clinical course of 20 891 patients with suspected acute myocardial infarction randomised between alteplase and streptokinase with or without heparin, *Lancet* (1990) **336**:71–5.

**3.** Horton R, tPA fast by GUSTO, *Lancet* (1993) **341**:1188.

**4.** Grines CL, Browne KF, Marco J et al, A comparison of immediate angioplasty with thrombolytic therapy for acute myocardial infarction, *N Engl J Med* (1993) **328**:673–9.

**5.** Zijlstra F, de Boer MJ, Hoorntje JCA et al, A comparison of immediate coronary angioplasty with intravenous streptokinase in acute myocardial infarction, *N Engl J Med* (1993) **328**:680–4.

**6.** Ulutin O, Balkur-Ulutin S, Ugur MS et al, The pharmacology and clinical pharmacology of defibrotide, a new profibrinolytic, antithrombotic, and antiplatelet substance, *Adv Exp Med Biol* (1990) **281**:429–38.

**7.** Fareed J, Wlenda JH, Iyer L, Hoppenstaedt S, Pifarre R, An objective perspective on recombinant hirudin, a new anticoagulant and antithrombotic agent, *Blood Coag Fibrinol* (1991) **2**:135–47.

**8.** MacMahon S, Sharpe N. Long–term antiplatelet therapy for the prevention of vascular disease, *Med J Aust* (1991) **154**:477–80.

**9.** Peto R, Gray R, Collins R, Randomised trial of prophylactic daily aspirin in British male doctors, *Br Med J* (1988) **296**:313–16.

**10.** Steering Committee of the Physicians' Health Study Research Group, Final report on the aspirin component of the ongoing physicians' health study, *N Engl J Med* (1989) **321**:129–35.

**11.** Horton RC, Kendall MJ, Aspirin in the next decade, *J Clin Pharmacol Ther* (1989) **14**:249–61.

**12.** RISC Group, Risk of myocardial infarction and death during treatment with low dose aspirin and intravenous heparin in men with unstable coronary artery disease, *Lancet* (1990) **336**:827–30.

**13.** Lewis MD, Davis IW, Archibald DG, Protective effects of aspirin against acute myocardial infarction and death in men with unstable angina, *N Engl J Med* (1983) **309**:396–403.

**14.** Cairns J, Gent M, Singer J, Aspirin, sulfinpyrazone or both in unstable angina, *N Engl J Med* (1985) **313**:1369–75.

**15.** Theroux P, Ouimet H, McCans J, Aspirin, heparin, or both to treat acute unstable angina, *N Engl J Med* (1988) **319**:1105–11.

**16.** Neriserneri GG, Gensini GF, Poggesi L et al, Effect of heparin, aspirin, or alteplase in reduction of myocardial ischaemia in refractory unstable angina, *Lancet* (1990) **335**:615–18.

**17.** Editorial, Aspirin after myocardial infarction, *Lancet* (1980) **i**:1172–3.

**18.** Persantin Aspirin Reinfarction Study Research Group, Persantin and aspirin in coronary heart disease, *Circulation* (1980) **62**:449–61.

**19** Persantin Aspirin Reinfarction Study Research Group, Secondary coronary prevention with persantin and aspirin, *J Am Coll Cardiol* (1986) **7**:251–69.

**20.** Antiplatelet Trialists' Collaboration, Secondary prevention of vascular disease by prolonged antiplatelet treatment, *Br Med J* (1988) **296**:320–31.

**21.** ISIS-II Collaborative Group, Randomised trial of intravenous streptokinase, oral aspirin, both, or neither among 17 187 cases of suspected acute myocardial infarction: ISIS II, *Lancet* (1988) **ii**:349–60.

**22.** AIMS Trial Study Group, Long-term effects of intravenous anistreplase in acute myocardial infarction: final report of the AIMS study, *Lancet* (1990) **335**:427–31.

**23.** Schreiber TL, Miller DH, Silvasi D et al, Superiority of warfarin over aspirin long–term after thrombolytic therapy for acute myocardial infarction, *Am Heart J* (1990) **119**:1238–44.

**24.** Report of the Sixty Plus Reinfarction Study Research Group, A double blind trial to assess long–term oral anticoagulant therapy in elderly patients after myocardial infarction, *Lancet* (1980) **ii**:989–93.

**25.** Smith P, Arnesen A, Holme I, The effect of warfarin on mortality and reinfarction after myocardial infarction, *N Engl J Med* (1990) **323**:147–52.

**26.** Ridker PM, Manson JE, Gasiano JM, Buring JE, Hennekens CH, Low-dose aspirin therapy for chronic stable angina: a randomised placebo-controlled clinical trial, *Ann Intern Med* (1991) **114**:835–9.

**27.** Manson JE, Stampfer MJ, Colditz GA et al, A prospective study of aspirin use and primary prevention of cardiovascular disease in women, *JAMA* (1991) **266**:521–7.

**28.** Meade TW, Roderick PJ, Bremnan PJ et al, Extracranial bleeding and other symptoms due to low-dose aspirin and low-intensity oral anticoagulation, *Thromb Haemost* (1992) **68**:1–6.

**29.** Lowe GDO, Laboratory investigation of pre-thrombotic states. In: Poller L, Thomson JM eds., Thrombosis and its management (Churchill Livingstone: Edinburgh 1993).

# Chapter 5
# **Arrhythmias**

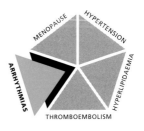

Sudden death is an important cause of both early and late mortality among patients with ischaemic heart disease. For example, about 50 per cent of all deaths among patients discharged from hospital after a myocardial infarction (MI) occur suddenly.[1] A substantial proportion of these deaths are the result of ventricular tachyarrhythmias.

An important question for the clinician faced with a patient who either has risk factors for ischaemic heart disease or has already had an index ischaemic event is: what is the best cardio-protective regimen available to prevent sudden death?

Although the electrophysiology of ventricular arrhythmias has been studied intensively during recent decades, and despite a clear rationale for intervention, unequivocal guidelines for preventing or reducing the risk of sudden death have yet to emerge. Indeed, the use of anti-arrhythmic drugs to reduce the incidence of sudden death has been an embarrassing and perplexing failure. What lessons can be drawn from the mass of disappointing evidence so far produced?

## ■ CAST AND BEYOND

Based on the Cardiac Arrhythmia Pilot Study,[2] encainide, flecainide, and moricizine were selected as drugs for full investigation in over 4000 patients randomized into the Cardiac Arrhythmia Suppression Trial (CAST).[3] After an MI, starting with an initial open-label phase to achieve adequate (about 80 per cent) suppression of the arrhythmia in question, patients were randomized either to one of these three agents or to placebo, and each was subsequently followed to see if there was a reduction in the incidence of sudden cardiac death. Most patients enrolled into CAST had frequent ventricular premature beats only.

Following a mean interval of 10 months, interim analysis revealed a statistically significant increase in mortality among patients receiving flecainide or encainide (7.7 per cent) compared with placebo (3.0 per cent). The pro-arrhythmic effects of these drugs seemed to be the cause of this result and a further report on the CAST data confirmed this belief by indicating the precise causes of death (Table 5.1).[4] Most

| | Arrhythmia | Non–arrhythmic cardiac causes | Non-cardiac causes |
|---|---|---|---|
| Drug[a] | 43 | 17 | 3 |
| Placebo | 16 | 5 | 5 |
| Total | 59 | 22 | 8 |

[a]Encainide or flecainide.

**Table 5.1** Causes of death in CAST.

non-arrhythmic cardiac deaths were attributable to either acute infarction with shock or a chronic history of coronary heart disease. Moreover, these adverse effects were more pronounced in older age groups.[5]

The message of CAST is clear – that, at best, physicians need to invoke a higher threshold for antiarrhythmic therapy when treating benign or potentially lethal ventricular arrhythmias, or that, at worst, there is no proven indication for the use of class IC antiarrhythmic drugs post-MI. Yet the patients most at risk are those who have had an episode of sustained ventricular fibrillation or ventricular tachycardia. No placebo-controlled trials have been done in this group alone.

A meta-analysis of 10 randomized controlled trials of all type I antiarrhythmic drugs in the prevention of sudden cardiac death after an MI strengthened the findings of the CAST investigators.[6] There was a tendency towards an adverse effect on mortality in the treated group. The trial drugs included members of all three subcategories of Vaughan Williams class I agents: IA, procainamide, aprindine; IB, phenytoin, tocainide, mexiletine, imipramine; IC, encainide, flecainide, moricizine. A combination of pro-arrhythmic effects, negative inotropism and interference with normal conduction are all likely to be possible causal mechanisms. Unselective treatment with antiarrhythmic therapy of patients post-MI remains unwarranted.

To replace the failed theories of past years, we need to revise our beliefs about arrhythmias in order to generate new paradigms for future research and to better understand what knowledge we already have.

European Task Force on antiarrhythmic drug therapy has offerred a radical reappraisal of long-held notions on drug classification and approaches to treatment.[7] They adopted a chess-like analogy to solve the complex clinical questions raised by the patient who presents with an arrhythmia.

The Vaughan Williams classification scheme (Table 5.2) of antiarrhythmic drugs has dominated thinking about therapy for two decades. However, the Task Force identified several important difficulties with this system: the hybrid mix of ion channel and receptor blockade; the exclusion of classes of antiarrhythmic drug that might activate receptors or channels; the exclusion of proven antiarrhythmic agents (adenosine, digoxin) that did not fit into the existing classes; the lack of a classification scheme according to the effects of drugs on diseased tissue; the failure of Vaughan Williams categories to acknowledge the multiple effects of some agents; and the oversimplistic nature of its format in the light of new evidence. All of these serve to diminish the relevance of the Vaughan Williams model.

The Task Force identified a series of 'vulnerable parameters' on the basis of the mechanism of arrhythmia generation. Each of these parameters is associated with an ionic current that may form a basis for pharmacological manipulation by focusing on a cellular mechanism or a molecular target. In Table 5.3, mechanism and variable parameter are equated and an example of an arrhythmia is linked to each.

Automaticity is the phenomenon of spontaneous impulse generation and can be enhanced during adrenergic stimulation; abnormal automaticity can result within damaged cardiac muscle fibres. The characteristic feature of cells that possess the property of automaticity is the presence of a slow decrease in the membrane potential during diastole (phase 4) (Figure 5.1), such that the membrane potential reaches threshold. Triggered activity develops as a result of afterdepolarizations that may interrupt the repolarization process (early afterdepolarizations) or which may take place after completion of repolarization (late afterdepolarizations). Re-entry mechanisms are common in an ischaemic myocardium that is characterized by irregular islands of viable tissue living amid regions of infarction. Circus movements are generated because of these areas of differential conduction velocity, and potentially lethal arrhythmias can be

| | Class 1 | Class II | Class III | Class IV |
|---|---|---|---|---|
| **Mechanism** | Direct membrane action; sodium channel blockade | Inhibition of sympathetic influences | Prolongation of repolarization | Calcium channel blockade |
| **Examples** | **IA** Quinidine<br>Procainamide<br>Disopyramide<br><br>**IB** Lignocaine<br>Phenytoin<br>Mexiletine<br><br>**IC** Flecainide<br>Encainide<br>Propafenone | Beta blockers | Bretylium<br>Amiodarone<br>Sotalol | Verapamil<br>Diltiazem |

**Table 5.2** Vaughan Williams classification of antiarrhythmic drugs.

| Mechanism | Vulnerable parameter | Examples |
|---|---|---|
| Automaticity | | |
| Enhanced normal automacity | Phase IV depolarization | Idiopathic VT |
| Abnormal automacity | Maximum diastolic potential or phase IV depolarization | Ectopic atrial tachycardia |
| Triggered activity | | |
| Early afterdepolarizations (EAD) | Action potential duration or EAD | Torsades de pointes |
| Delayed afterdepolarizations (DAD) | Calcium overload or DAD | Digoxin-induced arrhythmias |
| Sodium channel-dependent re-entry primary impaired conduction | Excitability and conduction | Sustained monomorphic VT |
| Conduction encroaching on refractoriness | Effective refractory period | Atrial fibrillation sustained polymorphic VT, VF |
| Calcium channel-dependent re-entry | Excitability and conduction | AV nodal re-entrant tachycardia |

**Table 5.3**  The Sicilian Gambit approach to arrhythmias.

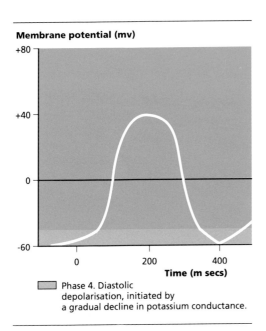

**Figure 5.1**
Cardiac action potential (sino-atrial node cell).

**Membrane potential (mv)**

Phase 4. Diastolic depolarisation, initiated by a gradual decline in potassium conductance.

initiated. Most clinically relevant arrhythmias are based on re-entry processes.

This diversion into a more mechanistic approach to arrhythmias illustrates how a systematic view of therapy could be achieved in the future. Each arrhythmia–mechanism–variable–parameter complex has a theoretical target for drug therapy. Rather than using an outmoded drug classification scheme to aid therapeutic decision-making, one will be able to adopt a patho-physiological method for the testing of new or existing drugs. The objections raised against the Vaughan Williams classification in the preceding discussion are largely overcome with the Sicilian Gambit.

Of course, as the Task Force noted, it is unreasonable to expect clinicians to commit Table 5.3 to memory. Nevertheless, the broad categories of *automaticity*, *triggered activity* and *re-entry* are

simple to understand and, together with conventional drug classification schemes, provide a rational basis for planning treatment
policy. In addition, this system helps to achieve an understanding about the how and why of arrhythmias rather than simply
promoting what at times can seem a rather random approach to
therapy. Yet this remains for the future. For now, how does the
clinician decide on what cardioprotective drug to use and when
to use it?

## ■ RISK STRATIFICATION

Some estimation of risk is crucial to decision-making on whether
to institute antiarrhythmic drug therapy. For example, the CAST
data showed that successful treatment of ventricular premature
beats, irrespective of their frequency and multiformity, is not
associated with a reduced risk of sudden death. Yet, after an MI,
although non-sustained ventricular tachycardia does increase the
risk of sudden death, no randomized controlled trial data are
available to support treatment.

Few well-designed trials have been done to investigate issues
of safety and efficacy. Most studies involve small numbers of
patients, arrhythmias are often poorly documented, dose titra-
tion to suppress the arrhythmia frequently does not take place,
and the duration of follow-up can be too brief to draw reliable
conclusions.

Moreover, the substantial side-effect profiles of antiarrhythmic
drugs produce a therapeutic equation heavily biased against
treatment. Amiodarone, in particular, has an array of adverse
reactions, including pulmonary infiltrates and fibrosis, thyroid
dysfunction, hepatitis, testicular dysfunction, neuropathies,
myopathies and even hypercholesterolaemia,[8] which discourage
widespread use of what is otherwise perceived to be an effective
antiarrhythmic agent.

Tolerance is further compromised if the patient has congestive
heart failure or left ventricular dysfunction, or is elderly.
Worsening of an existing arrhythmia (increased frequency, rate
or duration) or development of a new arrhythmia that is more
difficult to treat are additional pro-arrhythmic consequences of

drug therapy. For instance, CAST showed that the excess mortality from sudden death among patients treated with flecainide or encainide was about 5 per cent annually. Most antiarrhythmic drugs also have negative inotropic properties than can worsen or precipitate heart failure in up to 10 per cent of patients.

It would be easy to dismiss as hopelessly idealistic the notion of a cardioprotective drug regimen to prevent death from ischaemic-related arrhythmias. But accurate risk–benefit analysis depends on the background rate of sudden death in the population under study. The higher the mortality, as predicted by risk-factor assessment, the greater the benefit that treatment is likely to have. Here is a way forward.

The four main risk factors that can be assessed non-invasively are

- Symptoms
- Underlying heart disease
- Left ventricular dysfunction
- Type of arrhythmia

Some observers would also include the presence of absence of late potentials in a signal-averaged electrocardiogram.[9,10] For symptoms, loss of consciousness is especially associated with a high mortality rate. If underlying structural heart disease is present (e.g. after an MI), the incidence of sudden death is between 4 per cent and 8 per cent in the first year. Finally, arrhythmias can be broadly classified into benign, prognostically important (i.e. potentially malignant) and malignant. Sustained ventricular tachycardia and ventricular fibrillation fall into the latter category.

The difficulty with identifying these risk factors is that, although they are reasonably sensitive, they are non-specific and have high false-positive rates. This factor explains the CAST findings – the assignment of ventricular premature beats to a prognostically important class of arrhythmias wrongly placed enrolled patients into a high-risk group.

Combinations of non-invasive markers may thus be the answer, albeit at a loss in sensitivity. Patients with an annual risk of death approaching 10–20 per cent could then be identified. For now, a consensus of uncertainty should not induce a state of prescribing paralysis in the clinician. A careful search for the above four risk factors will help to give a firm foundation for treatment. There is ample evidence to support the view that cardioprotection is possible in these high-risk patients.

# ■ TREATMENT

The aims of any intervention are to alleviate symptoms that can be clearly linked to an arrhythmia and to prevent sudden cardiac death.

## ☐ Pharmacological intervention

Patients with hypertension are at risk of developing arrhythmias. Ghali et al[11] found that the degree of left ventricular hypertrophy in patients with hypertension and normal coronary arteries was directly correlated with the risk and severity of ventricular arrhythmias. This relationship was a continuous one: for every 1 mm increase in the thickness of the interventricular septum or posterior wall, there was a 2–3-fold increase in the occurrence and complexity of ventricular arrhythmias. Electrophysiological evidence supports a connection between left ventricular hypertrophy, ventricular arrhythmias and sudden death.[12]

Although data from clinical trials are conflicting,[13] the Metoprolol Atherosclerosis Prevention in Hypertensives (MAPHY) study showed a significant reduction in sudden deaths among patients treated with this lipophilic beta-blocker.[14] However, the MAPHY data may be considered as a subgroup of a larger trial, the Heart Attack Prevention in Hypertension Study (HAPPHY),[15] and so may only give an indication of efficacy. The HAPPHY trial result was inconclusive for the beta-blocker-treated group and thus firm conclusions about metoprolol cannot be drawn. But the hypothesis that in primary prevention trials a lipophilic beta-blocker can prevent sudden cardiac deaths needs further testing urgently.

Left ventricular hypertrophy is a structural response to high intravascular pressures. Antihypertensive treatment can reverse this structural damage to the heart.[16] Several classes of drug are effective: calcium antagonists, ACE inhibitors and beta-blockers (not diuretics). However, no study has yet correlated regression of left ventricular hypertrophy with beneficial effects on sudden death.

Recent work has emphasized the importance of cardiac sympathetic nervous activity in the generation of ventricular arrhythmias and sudden cardiac death. Meredith et al[17] found that rates of total noradrenaline spillover were 50 per cent higher (450 per cent higher for cardiac noradrenaline spillover) among patients who had had a spontaneously sustained episode of ventricular tachycardia or ventricular fibrillation compared with those without a history of ventricular arrhythmias. They concluded that there was selective activation of cardiac sympathetic nerves, probably caused by left ventricular dysfunction.

The only class of antiarrhythmic drugs that has shown convincing efficacy in the prevention of sudden death post-MI is beta-blockers.[18] Singh notes that 3 months of treatment with a beta-blocker that is started 4–28 days after an acute infarction reduces sudden cardiac death by 18–39 per cent. The average reduction in sudden death is about 30 per cent.[19] Beta-blockers seem to exert their effects by virtue of beta-blockade itself rather than suppression of ventricular premature beats. Not only is the threshold for ventricular arrhythmias raised, but also the heart rate is reduced and it is this variable that seems to be the key to understanding the benefits of beta-blockade. Drugs with intrinsic sympathomimetic activity, e.g. oxprenolol and pindolol, have little effect on mortality.

Concern about class Ic agents after CAST led to a switch in interest to other class I compounds. However, a meta-analysis of trials that have investigated the efficacy of quinidine found a statistically significant increased risk of death compared with flecainide, mexiletine, tocainide, and propafenone.[20] Clearly, the adverse effect of Ic drugs is a general property of the class as a whole and supposedly prognostically important arrhythmias should not routinely be treated with these agents.

Calcium-channel blockade, although theoretically appealing, is of no benefit in preventing sudden death and may even lead to a small increase in risk.[21]

Efficacy in preventing sudden death seems to reside in drugs that have no or only limited effects on cardiac conduction. For instance, amiodarone antagonizes sympathetic mechanisms and, in a prospective randomized study, significantly reduced mortality compared with untreated controls.[22] Individualized therapy with a range of other antiarrhythmics had no effect on rates of sudden death, although premature ventricular beats were suppressed. The antiarrhythmic drug evaluation group studied the benefits and risks of amiodarone, flecainide and propafenone in 141 patients with complex ventricular arrhythmias and cardiac disease.[23] After 2 years of various combinations of drug treatment, the median exposure to amiodarone was higher than that for flecainide and propafenone, suggesting a significantly better response to amiodarone. Because of amiodarone's side-effects, it cannot routinely be given. But, as Singh notes, the therapeutic and research emphasis 'must shift from antiarrhythmic agents that delay conduction to those that exert antifibrillatory actions by sympathetic antagonism and those that prolong refractoriness in cardiac muscle'.[18]

An alternative approach to individualized antiarrhythmic treatment might be to select a drug on the basis of invasive electrophysiological testing. Steinbeck et al[24] prospectively randomized patients with arrhythmias that were inducible by programmed electrical stimulation to either electrophysiologically guided drug therapy based on serial testing or metoprolol. After a mean follow-up of 2 years, there was no difference between the two groups in rates of symptomatic arrhythmia or sudden death.

In conclusion, prognostically important arrhythmias in combination with other risk factors – symptoms and degree of coexisting heart disease – should be treated with a beta-blocker that has no intrinsic sympathomimetic activity. The presentation of a malignant arrhythmia on a background of ischaemic heart disease necessitates treatment with a beta-blocker and/or a class I agent. Because of its toxicity, amiodarone should be reserved as a third-line agent in patients who are contraindicated from receiving beta-blockers, such as those with heart failure or reversible airways disease.[25,26] If patients have symptoms but no evidence of malignant arrhythmia, a beta-blocker only is indicated. A summary of these influences is shown in Figure 5.2.

## ☐ Non–pharmacological intervention

Apart from drugs, non-pharmacological means of preventing sudden death should be considered for symptomatic patients with severe underlying cardiac disease and a history of malignant

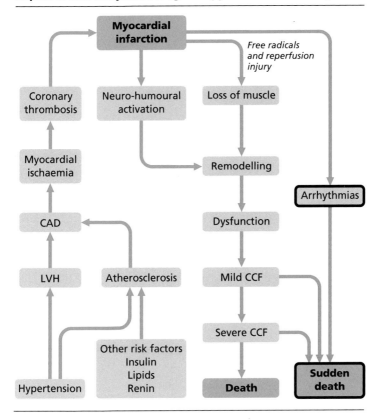

**Figure 5.2** Impact of antiarrhythmic drug therapy on the ischaemic cycle.

arrhythmias. The three main methods of treatment are surgery, catheter ablation and antitachycardia pacemakers (implantable defibrillators).

Surgery is intended to break the re-entry circuit[27] but has been largely replaced by newer techniques. Radiofrequency current catheter ablation overcomes the complications of direct-current shock and has been successfully reported by several groups.[28–30] In addition, the notion of a targetable tachycardia-related artery has received support from studies where ethanol has been injected to elicit permanent damage to an arrhythmogenic area.[31] Finally, the implantable defibrillator offers the ultimate treatment of a fatal arrhythmia – immediate abortion of fibrillation.[32] For patients refractory to drug therapy, this device is the best and most reliable antiarrhythmic treatment available. Third-generation implantable cardioverter defibrillators with antitachycardia pacing will offer many more patients both symptomatic and survival benefit.[33] Several trials, such as the Multicenter Automatic Defibrillator Implantation Trial (MADIT) and the Multicenter Unsustained Tachycardia Trial (MUSST), will settle these uncertainties during the next few years.

## References

**1.** Rosenthal ME, Sudden cardiac death following acute myocardial infarction, *Am Heart J* (1985) 109:865–76.

**2.** CAPS Investigators, The cardiac arrhythmia pilot study, *Am J Cardiol* (1986) **57**:91–5.

**3.** Cardiac Arrhythmia Suppression Trial (CAST) Investigators Preliminary Report, Effect of encainide and flecainide on mortality in a randomised trial of arrhythmia suppression after myocardial infarction, *N Engl J Med* (1989) **321**:406–11.

**4.** Echt DS, Liebson PR, Mitchell B et al, Mortality and morbidity in patients receiving encainide, flecainide, or placebo: the Cardiac Arrhythmia Suppression Trial, *N Engl J Med* (1991) **324**:781–8.

**5.** Akiyama T, Pawitan Y, Campbell WB et al, Effects of advancing age on the efficacy and side effects of anti-arrhythmic drugs in post myocardial infarction patients with ventricular arrhythmias: the CAST investigators, *J Am Geriatr Soc* (1992) **40**:666–72.

**6.** Hine LK, Laird NM, Hewitt P, Chalmers TC, Meta-analysis of empirical long-term antiarrhythmic therapy after myocardial infarction, *JAMA* (1989) **262**:3037–40.

**7.** Task Force of the Working Group on Arrhythmias of the European Society of Cardiology, The Sicilian Gambit – a new approach to the classification of antiarrhythmic drugs based on their actions on arrhythmogenic mechanisms, *Eur Heart J* (1991) **12**:1112–31.

**8.** Wiersinga WM, Trip MD, Van Beeren MH, Plomp TA, Oosting H, An increase in plasma cholesterol independent of thyroid function during long-term amiodarone therapy: a dose-dependent relationship, *Ann Intern Med* (1991) **114**:128–32.

**9.** Dennis AR, Richards DA, Cody DV et al, Prognostic significance of ventricular tachycardia and fibrillation induced at programmed stimulation and delayed potentials detected on the signal-averaged electrocardiograms of survivors of acute myocardial infarction, *Circulation* (1986) **74**:731–45.

**10.** Gomes JA, Winters SL, Ergin A et al, Clinical and electrophysiological determinants, treatment and survival of patients with sustained malignant ventricular tachyarrhythmias occurring late after myocardial infarction, *J Am Coll Cardiol* (1991)**17**:320–6.

**11.** Ghali JK, Kadakia S, Cooper RS, Liao Y, Impact of left ventricular hypertrophy on ventricular arrhythmias in the absence of coronary artery disease, *J Am Coll Cardiol* (1991) **17**:1277–82.

**12.** Messerti FH, Grodzicki T, Hypertension, left ventricular hypertrophy, ventricular arrhythmias and sudden death, *Eur Heart J* (1992) **13** (suppl D):66–69.

**13.** Kendall MJ, *Beta blockade and cardioprotection* (Science Press: London, 1991).

**14.** Olsson G, Tuomilehto J, Berglund G et al, Primary prevention of sudden cardiovascular death in hypertensive patients, *Am J Hypertens* (1991) **4**:151–8.

**15.** Wilhelmsen L, Berglund G, Elmfeldt D et al, Beta blockers versus diuretics in hypertensive men: main results from the HAPPHY trial, *J Hypertens* (1987) **5**:561–72.

**16.** Novo S, Abrignani MG, Corda M, Strano A, Cardiovascular structural changes in hypertension: possible regression during long term antihypertensive treatment, *Eur Heart J* (1991) **12** (suppl G):47–52.

**17.** Meredith IT, Broughton A, Jennings GL, Esler MD, Evidence of a selective increase in cardiac sympathetic activity in patients with sustained ventricular arrhythmias, *N Engl J Med* (1991) **325**:618–24.

**18.** Singh BN, Advantages of beta blockers versus antiarrhythmic agents and calcium antagonists in secondary prevention after myocardial infarction, *Am J Cardiol* (1990) **66**:9C–20C.

**19.** Yusuf S, Peto R, Lewis J, Collins R, Sleight P, Beta blockade during and after myocardial infarction: an overview of the randomised trials, *Prog Cardiovasc Dis* (1985) **27**:335–71.

**20.** Morganroth J, Goin JE, Quinidine-related mortality in the short-to-medium-term treatment of ventricular arrhythmias: a meta-analysis, *Circulation* (1991) **84**:1977–83.

**21.** Yusuf S, Forberg CD, Effects of calcium channel blockers on survival after acute myocardial infarction, *Cardiovasc Drugs Ther* (1987) **1**:343–44.

**22.** Burkart F, Pfisterar M, Kiowski W, Burckhardt D, Follath D, Improved survival of patients with symptomatic ventricular arrhythmias after myocardial infarction with amiodarone, *Circulation* (1989) **80**:110–19.

**23.** Anti-arrhythmic Drug Evaluation Group, A multicentre, randomised trial on the benefit/risk profile of amiodarone, flecainide, and propafenone in patients with cardiac disease and complex ventricular arrhythmias, *Eur Heart J* (1992) **13**:1251–8.

**24.** Steinbeck G, Andresen D, Bach P et al, A comparison of electrophysiologically guided antiarrhythmic drug therapy with beta-blocker therapy in patients with symptomatic sustained ventricular tachyarrhythmias, *N Engl J Med* (1992) **327**:987–92.

**25.** Buckhardt D, Hoffman A, Kiowski W, Pfisterer M, Burkart F, Effect of antiarrhythmic therapy on mortality after myocardial infarction, *J Cardiovasc Pharmacol* (1991) **17** (suppl 6): 77–81.

**26.** Gill J, Heel RC, Fitton A, Amiodarone: an overview of its pharmacological properties, and review of its therapeutic use in cardiac arrhythmias, *Drugs* (1992) **43**:69–110.

**27.** Lawrie GM, Pacifico A, Kaushik R, Nahas C, Earle N, Factors predictive of results of direct ablative operations for drug-refractory ventricular tachycardia, *J Thorac Cardiovasc Surgery* (1991) **101**:44–5.

**28.** Yeung-Lai-Wah JA, Alison JF, Lonergan L et al, High success rate of atrioventricular node ablation with radiofrequency energy, *J Am Coll Cardiol* (1991) **18**:1753–8.

**29.** Wiwano S, Aizawa Y, Satoh M, Chinushi M, Shibata A, Low energy catheter electrical ablation for sustained ventricular tachycardia, *Am Heart J* (1991) **122**:81–8.

**30.** Lesh MD, Van Hare GF, Schamp DJ et al, Curative percutaneous catheter ablation using radiofrequency energy for accessory pathways in all locations: results in 100 consecutive patients, *J Am Coll Cardiol* (1992) **19**:1303–9.

**31.** Brugada P, de Swart J, Smeets JLRM, Wellens HJJ, Termination of tachycardias by interrupting blood supply to the arrhythmogenic area, *Am J Cardiol* (1988) **62**:387–92.

**32.** Mirowski M, Reid DR, Mower MM et al, Termination of malignant ventricular arrhythmias with an implanted automatic defibrillator in human beings, *N Engl J Med* (1980) **303**:322–4.

**33.** Cannon DS, A critical appraisal of indications for the implantable cardioverter defibrillator (ICD), *Clin Cardiol* (1992) **15**:369–72.

# Chapter 6
# **Menopause**

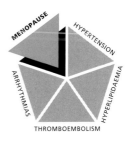

Women have fared badly in the hands of those who investigate cardiovascular disease. Cardiac-related deaths are the leading cause of mortality among women who live in industrialized countries, and especially so in postmenopausal women, yet only a fraction of the total studies done on heart disease have been directed at women.[1] Perhaps this research bias is because the risk of a younger woman developing coronary heart disease is substantially less than in a man: premenopausal women have only 20 per cent of the coronary mortality of men. But if this reason is correct, it ignores the overall toll that coronary disease exacts on women.

Over 50 per cent of postmenopausal women die from cardiovascular causes; half of these deaths are related to coronary heart disease and 80 per cent are in women aged below 65 years. The Framingham study showed that the incidence of myocardial infarction among women after the menopause rose rapidly towards that of men (Figure 6.1).[2] Oestrogens have profound effects on lipoprotein metabolism and are thought to

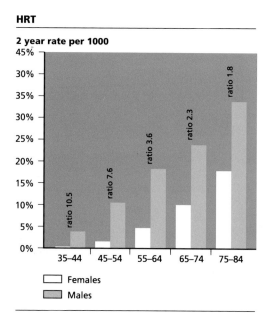

**HRT**

**2 year rate per 1000**

**Figure 6.1**
Incidence of myocardial infarction by age and sex.[2]

have striking cardioprotective actions. Women who have had an oophorectomy are twice as likely to develop coronary heart disease.[3]

Two questions naturally arise. First, what is the evidence that oestrogens have any effect on the risk of cardiovascular disease? Second, what cardiovascular data are there to support replacing oestrogen in women with declining ovarian function?

# ■ EFFECTS OF HORMONE REPLACEMENT THERAPY ON CARDIOVASCULAR RISK FACTORS

Oestrogens may exert their effects on the cardiovascular system in one or more of several ways. For instance, oestrogens have:

- beneficial effects on lipoprotein metabolism
- direct actions on vascular tone
- effects on mediators that influence vascular function
- effects on the microcirculation[4]

## ☐ Lipoprotein metabolism

About 30–50 per cent of the effects of oestrogen can be attributed to their effects on lipoproteins.[5] The menopause is associated with both quantitative and qualitative effects on lipoprotein profiles. After the menopause, women have significant reductions in HDL cholesterol with concomitant increases in LDL cholesterol,[6] and these persist after controlling for age, smoking and body-mass index. Cross-sectional studies confirm increased LDL cholesterol concentrations among postmenopausal women,[7] who also have higher quantities of small, dense (atherogenic) LDL particles than their premenopausal counterparts.[8]

Hormone replacement therapy modifies the lipoprotein profile by shifting it towards its original premenopausal state. Different formulations have profoundly different effects on lipid metabolism. For example, Haarbo and co-workers randomized otherwise healthy early postmenopausal women to four treatments and two placebo groups.[9] Treatment consisted of 2 mg oestradiol (O) either sequentially combined with 75 µg levonorgestrel (O/LNG), 10 mg medroxyprogesterone acetate (O/MPA) or 150 µg desorgestreal (O/DG), *or* constinuously combined with 1 mg cyproterone acetate (O/CPA). After 84 days of treatment, all treatment regimes had reduced LDL cholesterol significantly:

| | |
|---|---|
| O/LNG | 10.9 per cent |
| O/MPA | 14.4 per cent |
| O/DG | 10.7 per cent |
| O/CPA | 6 per cent |

There was no significant change in HDL cholesterol concentration in any treatment group.

Walsh et al studied healthy and postmenopausal women who had normal lipid concentrations at baseline.[10] In their first protocol, conjugated oestrogens (0.625 mg and 1.25 mg per day) were compared with placebo for 3 months. In their second protocol, oral micronized oestradiol (2 mg per day) was compared with transdermal oestradiol (0.1 mg twice a week) and placebo for 6 weeks. In the first study, the low and high dose of oestradiol reduced mean LDL cholesterol concentration by 15 per cent and 19 per cent, respectively, and increased HDL cholesterol by 16 per cent and 18 per cent, respectively. VLDL triglyceride concentrations were increased by 24 per cent and 42 per cent, respectively. All of these changes were statistically significant. In their second study, oral oestradiol reduced LDL cholesterol concentrations by 14 per cent and increased HDL cholesterol concentration by 15 per cent. Transdermal oestradiol had no effect, thus confirming several previous reports.[11,12]

To summarize, oestrogen reduces LDL cholesterol, probably by augmenting its uptake into cells, and increases HDL cholesterol, probably by reducing the activity of hepatic lipoprotein lipase. By suppressing the activity of plasma lipoprotein lipase, oestrogen also causes serum triglyceride concentrations to rise. These changes are dose dependent. Since the liver is the principal regulator of LDL and HDL metabolism, drugs that avoid first-pass metabolism are likely to have only limited effects on lipoprotein profiles. However, more recent studies have been able to show a benefit of transdermal patches. For instance, Crook et al[13] found that transdermal preparations of continuous 17-beta-oestradiol or cyclic norethindrone acetate produced similar reductions in total and LDL cholesterol compared with oral continuous conjugated equine oestrogens. In addition, transdermal therapy led to falls in circulating triglycerides while this lipid fraction rose with oral hormone replacement.

Progestogens must be given with oestrogens in women who have not undergone a hysterectomy. About 33 per cent of women who take 0.625 mg of conjugated oestrogens develop endometrial hyperplasia; 20 per cent of these will develop endometrial carcinoma. However, progestogens have adverse effects on lipoprotein metabolism, which may counteract the beneficial effects of oestrogens. They promote HDL catabolism and diminish its synthesis. Hirvonen et al[14] showed a gradation in effects of progestogen on HDL cholesterol: natural progesterone had the least effect, followed by $C_{21}$ progestogens (medroxyprogesterone acetate and megestrol acetate), and finally by 19-nor-progestins (norethindrone and levonorgestrel). However, progestogens also reduce the total triglyceride concentration, thereby counterbalancing the rise produced by oestrogen therapy. Progestogens also seem to antagonize the beneficial effects of oestrogens on arterial wall prostacyclin production[15] and vascular tone.[16]

The issue over the risk–benefit equation for progestins has become clearer with the publication by Nabulsi et al[17] of a survey of metabolic variables among 4958 postmenopausal women. Four groups were studied: current users of oestrogen alone, current users of oestrogen and a progestin (mostly medroxyprogesterone acetate), non-users who had once received oestrogen, and non-users who had never received oestrogen.

All current users of oestrogen had higher circulating concentrations of HDL (both $HDL_2$ and $HDL_3$ subfractions) and apo A1 but lower concentrations of LDL, apo B, Lp(a), fibrinogen, antithrombin III, fasting glucose, and insulin (Figure 6.2). These differences translated into a 42 per cent potential reduction in risk of coronary heart disease, with the greatest benefit being found in women taking an oestrogen *and* progestin.

Progestins clearly differ from one another, especially in relation to their binding to androgen receptors. Thus, levonorgestrel (derived from testosterone) is more androgenic, and in some circumstances has more deleterious effects on serum lipids than other progestins.[18] Dydrogesterone also seems free of adverse lipid effects[19] and newer, third–generation progestins (e.g. desorgestrel, gestodene) may be even safer.

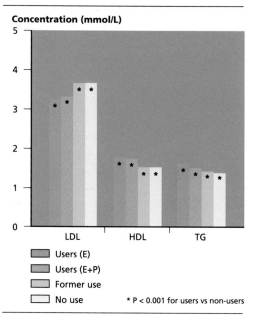

**Figure 6.2** The influence of oestrogens and progestins on lipid profiles in postmenopausal women. *$p < 0.001$ for users versus non-users.[17]

- Concentration (mmol/L) axis labels: 0, 1, 2, 3, 4, 5
- Groups: LDL, HDL, TG
- Users (E)
- Users (E+P)
- Former use
- No use

* $P < 0.001$ for users vs non-users

## ☐ Alternative mechanisms

What of the other 50–70 per cent of beneficial effect attributed to oestrogen? Oestrogens seem to improve blood flow (oestrogen receptors are found in vessel walls[20]) in several vascular beds but this effect may be opposed by the concurrent administration of progestogens.[21] Moreover, oestrogens increase circulating concentrations of prostacyclin ($PGI_2$, derived from endothelial cells and a powerful vasodilator with anti-platelet-adhesiveness activity) and decrease plasma thromboxane $A_2$ (derived from platelets, and with opposite actions to those of prostacyclin). Evidence also suggests that the arteries of post-menopausal women produce significantly less prostacyclin than pre-menopausal arteries.[22] The favourable prostacyclin/thromboxane balance induced by oestrogens may provide substantial protection against thrombosis. There seems to be no influence of oestrogen on Lp(a),[23] although Nabulsi et al[17] found significant differences between users and non-users of hormone replacement.

# ■ EVIDENCE OF CLINICAL BENEFIT

Much of medical practice is based on the wholly genuine belief that one's actions are likely to benefit a patient. Yet the dividing line between decision-making based on firm evidence and intervention based on myth is a fine one. When interpreting clinical trials, enthusiasts often let the forces of logic and rationality get the better of their judgement about data. Just as journalists hate to let truth get in the way of a good story, so doctors often persuade themselves that the evidence should not get in the way of their perfectly reasonable hypothesis.

And so it is with hormone replacement therapy (and, of course, with lipids). The rational arguments underpinning oestrogen replacement seem unassailable and we hope to have convinced you of their strength up to this point. But from now on, we are working in the absence of adequate clinical trial data.

Medical journals are littered with inconclusive retrospective case-control studies on the efficacy of hormone replacement. The inherent bias is great, the conclusions that one can draw are unreliable, and the data are largely misleading.

The next best thing to a randomized controlled trial is a prospective cohort study. These studies assume that women who take hormone replacement therapy and those who do not are the same. Regarding oestrogen replacement, four reports out of many merit particular discussion.[24-27]

Bush and co-workers[24] took data from the Lipid Research Clinics' Study after an average follow-up of 8.5 years. Oestrogen users and non-users had the same levels of health at enrollment, and a 40 per cent reduction in cardiovascular disease mortality was found among users. For those women who entered the study with pre-existing evidence of cardiac disease (12 per cent of the total), oestrogen replacement was associated with a 71 per cent reduction in cardiovascular deaths even after adjustment for smoking.

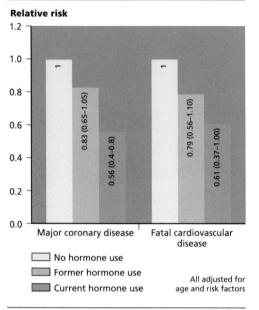

**Relative risk of cardiovascular disease among women who either formerly or were currently taking hormone replacement therapy (ref 25)**

Relative risk

1.2

1.0 — 1

0.8 — 0.83 (0.65–1.05)

0.6 — 0.56 (0.4–0.8)

0.4 —

0.2 —

0.0 —

Major coronary disease

1

0.79 (0.56–1.10)

0.61 (0.37–1.00)

Fatal cardiovascular disease

☐ No hormone use
☐ Former hormone use
■ Current hormone use

All adjusted for age and risk factors

**Figure 6.3** Ten-year follow-up from the Nurses' Health Study. All adjusted for age and risk factors.[25]

In a 10-year follow-up of over 48 000 postmenopausal women in the Nurse's Health Study (over 330 000 person years), the overall relative risk of major coronary disease among women taking oestrogen was 0.56 (95 per cent confidence interval 0.40–0.80) after adjusting for age and other cardiovascular risk factors (Figure 6.3).[25] The relative risk for cardiovascular mortality was 0.72 (0.55–0.95). There was no effect on the risk of stroke (0.97; 0.65–1.45) and the confidence interval for *total mortality* just reached 1 (0.89; 0.78–1.00). Therefore oestrogens roughly halved the risk of major or fatal cardiovascular disease but had no effect on total mortality, a finding supported by the Walnut Creek study (relative risk [total mortality] = 0.8; 95 per cent CI 0.6–1.1).[26] Those studies that have reported beneficial effects of hormone replacement therapy on total mortality[24,27] are generally agreed to be overestimates because women with existing disease were excluded from oestrogen treatment groups at entry.

Henderson and colleagues[27] examined the relation between hormone replacement and total mortality. After more than 7 years of follow-up, women with a history of oestrogen use had a 20 per cent lower age-adjusted, all-cause mortality than lifetime non-users. Current users who had taken oestrogen for 15 years or more had a 40 per cent reduction in their total mortality. The confounding variable in this analysis has already been pointed out, i.e. exclusion of women with existing coronary artery disease (CAD). Deaths from all categories of chronic arteriosclerotic and cerebrovascular disease were also reduced among those taking oestrogen.

In a quantitative overview of the cardiovascular effects of hormone replacement,[28] Stampfer and Colditz concluded that oestrogen treatment yielded an overall beneficial relative risk of 0.56 (0.50–0.61). When prospective cohort and angiographic studies only were considered, the summary relative risk for coronary heart disease was 0.50 (0.43–0.56).

The one large prospective study that initially failed to show a benefit from oestrogen replacement came from the Framingham cohort,[29] in which oestrogen users had an increased risk of coronary heart disease, defined as angina, myocardial infarction (MI), or sudden death. In a later publication,[30] angina was excluded from the analysis and the results were this time not adjusted for HDL cholesterol – fortunately for those committed to the notion of hormone replacement therapy, a significantly lower risk of cardiovascular disease was then found among women aged 50–59 who were taking oestrogen.

A further complication is how one deals with the variable of progestogen co-therapy. As we have noted, some progestogen preparations might reverse the beneficial effects of oestrogen – how does this concern translate into the epidemiological data so far available? The plain answer is that we do not know, although an observational study, in which 43 per cent of women were taking both oestrogen and progesterone, showed the same degree of protection as for those taking unopposed oestrogen.[31]

What is needed – and with some urgency – is a formal randomized controlled clinical trial with currently available oral combination hormone replacement preparations, transdermal patches, and newer agents (e.g. tibolone). Meade and Berra[32] have provided a convincing argument in favour of three possible protocols:

- Opposed versus unopposed oestrogen replacement in non-hysterectomized women
- Opposed versus unopposed oestrogen replacement in hysterectomized women
- Hormone replacement therapy (opposed for non-hysterectomized women, unopposed for hysterectomized women) versus no hormone replacement therapy.

A preliminary feasibility study[33] suggests that such trials, especially the second and third options, would receive strong support from those who would be responsible for recruiting patients.

## ■ RISKS OF HORMONE REPLACEMENT THERAPY

Why are so few women receiving hormone replacement therapy? The answer is that there is a widespread perception of increased risk for developing cancer.

The greatest concern is attached to the risk of breast cancer. Although oestrogens may be an important causal factor in carcinogenesis, the epidemiological surveys on risk of hormone replacement are contradictory. It is clear that short-term use of oestrogen (under 10 years) does not appreciably increase risk.[34] However, this same meta-analysis found that long-term (15 years or more) treatment with oestrogen was associated with a 30 per cent increased risk of breast cancer. Yet even meta-analyses are confusing. Dupont and Page found that the overall relative risk of developing breast cancer with hormone replacement was 1.07.[35] When factors such as dose and duration of treatment were taken into account, their results suggested that oestrogen replacement at a dose of 0.625 mg/day or less did not increase the risk of breast cancer.

Even if one accepts the possibility of an increased *incidence*, the risk of dying of breast cancer does not seem to be different. Bergquist and colleagues found that 5-year mortality rates among those taking oestrogens who developed breast cancer were significantly lower than in non-users with breast cancer (15 per cent versus 25 per cent).[36] Other reports substantiate the claim that the risk of dying from breast cancer in oestogren users is the same or even lower than in non-users.[27,37]

The risk of endometrial cancer has now been eliminated by giving at least 12 days of progestogens per cycle in women with an intact uterus. There is no significant association between hormone replacement therapy and ovarian cancer cervical cancer, or thromboembolism. Furthermore, the natural oestrogens contained in hormone replacement preparations do not increase blood pressure. Oestrogens do increase the possibility of gall bladder disease and they should probably be avoided in patients with a history of melanoma.[38]

## ■ CONCLUSIONS

Let us briefly review the facts (Figure 6.4):

- There is a strong rational case in favour of hormone replacement therapy as a means of preventing coronary mortality.
- Even if one limits oneself to the best available epidemiological studies, the case for a cardioprotective effect of oestrogen replacement seems proven.
- The excess risk of breast cancer up to 15 years is vanishingly small and, anyway, the risk of death from breast cancer is actually lower in those taking oestrogen replacement.
- Thus, for women who have undergone a hysterectomy, oral hormone replacement therapy with unopposed oestrogen will reduce cardiovascular mortality by up to 50 per cent.

There are two difficulties. First, this recommendation is not based on any truly experimental evidence (randomized intervention trials). Second, total mortality is consistently unaffected by hormone replacement. The best way to proceed, therefore, is

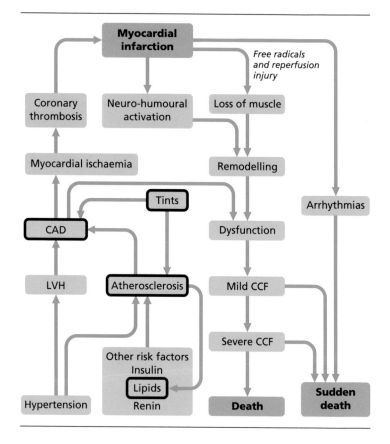

**Figure 6.4** Impact of hormone replacement therapy on the ischaemic cycle.

probably to offer the woman a choice based on these facts: her risk of cardiovascular disease will fall, but her overall risk of death will remain the same.

Of course, recommendations for treatment are not made on the basis of cardiovascular end-points alone. The beneficial effects of hormone replacement therapy on menopausal symptoms are clear and unambiguous. Moreover, oestrogen replacement slows or eliminates vertebral body and femoral neck bone loss, especially when given early in the menopause.[39] Epidemiological studies suggest that exogenous oestrogens lead to a 50 per cent reduction in the risk of hip fractures and osteoporotic fractures.

For non-hysterectomized women, the decision is more complex since the effects of the progesterone component are uncertain. Only prospective trials will settle this issue. In relation to the prevention of cardiovascular disease, physicians should not offer optimistic advice based either on what they *wished* the data would show or on what they hope future trials will reveal. Women deserve to be fully informed about the lack of data on both total mortality and effects of progestogens and involved in the choice about whether or not to opt for hormone replacement therapy. Ideally, one would be in a position to invite such women to take part in clinical trials.

## References

**1.** Khaw K-T, Where are the women in studies of coronary heart disease? *Br Med J* (1993) **306**:1145–6.

**2.** Lerner DJ, Kannel WB, Patterns of coronary disease morbidity and mortality: a 26 year follow-up of the Framingham population, *Am Heart J* (1986) **III**:383–90.

**3.** Colditz GA, Willett WC, Stampfer MJ et al, Menopause and the risk of coronary heart disease in women, *N Engl J Med* (1987) **316**:1105–10.

**4.** Sarrel P, Effects of ovarian steroids on the cardiovascular system. In: Ginsberg J, ed, *The circulation in the female from the cradle to the grave.* (Parthenon: Carnforth, 1989) 117.

**5.** Lobo RA, Effects of hormonal replacement on lipids and lipoproteins in postmenopausal women, *J Clin Endocrinol Metab* (1991) **73**:925–30.

**6.** Matthews KA, Meilahn E, Kuller LH et al, Menopause and risk factors for coronary heart disease, *N Engl J Med* (1989) **321**:641–6.

**7.** Knopp RH, Effects of estrogen on serum lipoproteins and significance or arteriosclerotic disease, *Chol Cor Dis* (1990) **2**:8–10.

**8.** Campos H, McNamara JR, Wilson DWF, Ordovas JM, Schaefer EJ, Differences in low density lipoprotein subfractions and apolipoproteins in premenopausal and postmenopausal women, *J Clin Endocrinol Metab* (1988) **67**:30–5.

**9** Haarbo J, Hassager C, Jensen SB, Riis BJ, Christiansen C, Serum lipids, lipoproteins, and apolipoproteins during postmenopausal estrogen replacement therapy combined with either 19-nortestosterone derivatives or 17-hydroxyprogesterone derivatives, *Am J Med* (1991) **90**:584–9.

**10.** Walsh BW, Schiff I, Rosner B et al,.Effects of postmenopausal estrogen replacement on the concentrations and metabolism of plasma lipoproteins, *N Engl J Med* (1991) **325**:1196–204.

**11.** Chetkowski RJ, Meldrum DR, Steingold KA et al, Biologic effects of transdermal estradiol, *N Engl J Med* (1986) **314**:1615–20.

**12.** Haas S, Walsh B, Evans S et al, The effect of transdermal estradiol on hormone and metabolic dynamics over a six-week period, *Obstet Gynecol* (1988) **71**:671–6.

**13.** Crook D, Cust MP, Gangar KF et al, Comparison of transdermal and oral oestrogen–progestin replacement therapy: effects on serum lipids and lipoproteins, *Am J Obstet Gynecol* (1992) **166**:950–5.

**14.** Hirvonen E, Malkonen M, Manninen V, Effects of different progestagens on lipoproteins during postmenopausal replacement therapy, *N Engl J Med* (1981) **304**:560–3.

**15.** Makila VM, Wahlberg L, Vlinikka L, Ylikorkala O, Regulation of prostacyclin and thromboxane production by human umbilical vessels: the effects of estradiol and progesterone in a superfusion model, *Prostaglandins Leukotrienes Med* (1982) **8**:115–24.

**16.** Yui Y, Aoyama T, Morishita H et al, Severn prostacyclin stabilizing factor is identical to apolipoprotein A-1 (apo A-1): a novel function of apo A-1, *J Clin Invest* (1988) **82**:803–4.

**17** Nabulsi AA, Folsom AR, White A et al, Association of hormone-replacement therapy with various cardiovascular risk factors in postmenopausal women, *N Engl J Med* (1993) **328**:1069–75.

**18.** Swartz DP (ed.), *Hormone replacement therapy* (Williams and Wilkins: Baltimore, 1992) 162–3.

**19.** Van der Mooren MJ, Demacker PN, Thomas CM, Rolland R, Beneficial effects on serum lipoproteins by 17-beta-oestradiol-dydrogesterone therapy in postmenopausal women: a prospective study, *Eur J Obstet Gynecol Reprod Biol* (1992) **47**:153–60.

**20.** McGill HC, Sex steroid hormone receptors in the cardiovascular system, *Postgrad Med* (1989) **85**: 64–68.

**21.** Bourne T, Hillard TC, Whitehead MI, Crook D, Oestrogens, arterial status, and postmenopausal women, *Lancet* (1990) **335**:1470–1.

**22.** Steinleitner A, Stanczyk FZ, Levin JH et al, Decreased in vitro production of 6–keto–prostaglandin $F_1$alpha by uterine arteries from postmenopausal women, *Am J Obstet Gynecol* (1989) **161**:1677–81.

**23.** Lobo RA, Notelovitz M, Bernstein L et al, Lp(a) lipoprotein: relationship to cardio-vascular disease risk factors, exercise, and estrogen, *Am J Obstet Gynecol* (1992) **166**:1182–90.

**24.** Bush TL, Barrett-Connor E, Cowan LD et al, Cardiovascular mortality and non-contraceptive estrogen use in women: results from the Lipid Research Clinics Program Follow-up Study, *Circulation* (1987) **75**:1002–8.

25. Stampfer MJ, Colditz GA, Willett WC et al, Post menopausal estrogen therapy and cardiovascular disease: ten-year follow-up from the Nurse's Health Study, *N Engl J Med* (1991) **325**:756–62.

**26.** Petitti DB, Perlman JA, Sidney S, Noncontraceptive estrogens and mortality: long-term follow-up of women in the Walnut Creek study, *Obstet Gynecol* (1987) **70**:289–93.

**27.** Henderson BE, Paganini-Hill A, Ross RK, Decreased mortality in users of estrogen replacement therapy, *Arch Intern Med* (1991) **151**:75–8.

**28.** Stampfer MJ, Colditz GA, Estrogen replacement therapy and coronary heart disease: a quantitative assessment of the epidemiologic evidence, *Prev Med* (1991) **20**;447–63.

**29.** Wilson PWF, Garrison RJ, Castelli WPP, Postmenopausal estrogen use, cigarette smoking, and cardiovascular morbidity in women over 50, *N Engl J Med* (1985) **313**:1038–43.

**30.** Eaker ED, Castelli WP, Coronary heart disease and its risk factors among women in the Framingham Study. In: Eaker E et al, eds, *Coronary heart disease in women.* (Haymarket Doyma: New York, 1987) 122–30.

**31.** Hunt K, Vessey M, Mcpherson K et al, Long-term surveillance of mortality and cancer incidence in women receiving hormone replacement therapy, *Br J Obstet Gynecol* (1987) **94**:620.

**32.** Meade TW, Berra A, Hormone replacement therapy and cardiovascular disease, *Br Med Bull* (1992) **48**:276–308.

**33.** Wilkes HC, Meade TW, Hormone replacement therapy in general practice: a survey of doctors in the MRC's General Practice Research Framework, *Br Med J* (1991) **302**:1317–20.

**34.** Steinberg KK, Thaker SB, Smith SJ et al, A meta-analysis of the effect of estrogen replacement therapy on the risk of breast cancer, *JAMA* (1991) **265**:1985–90.

**35.** Dupont WD, Page DL, Menopausal estrogen replacement therapy and breast cancer, *Arch Intern Med* (1991) **151**:67–72.

**36.** Bergquist L, Adami HO, Persson I, Bergstrom R, Prognosis after breast cancer diagnosis in women exposed to estrogen and estrogen-progestogen replacement therapy, *Am J Epidemiol* (1989) **130**:221–8.

**37.** Colditz GA, Stampfer MJ, Wilett WC et al, Prospective study of estrogen replacement therapy and risk of breast cancer in postmenopausal women, *JAMA* (1990) **264**:2648–53.

**38.** Whitcroft SIJ, Stevenson JL, Hormone replacement therapy: risks and benefits, *Clin Endocrinol* (1992) **36**:15–20.

**39.** Lindsay R, Prevention and treatment of osteoporosis, *Lancet* (1993) **341**:801–5.

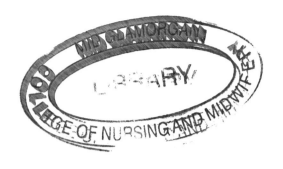

# Chapter 7
# The future of cardioprotection

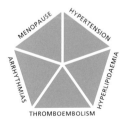

The tendency for medicine to progress in terms of the latest fashion is especially noticeable in cardiology. As the technical means for observing (angioscopy) and physically removing (laser angioplasty, rotablation) coronary atheroma have developed at a remarkable pace, so the notion that judicious pharmacological intervention alone can preserve myocardium and save lives has receded into relative obscurity. For instance, CAVEAT (the Coronary Angioplasty versus Excisional Atherectomy Trial)[1] is one of several studies comparing these different technologies, on the basis that removing atheroma from the artery is better than simply splitting the plaque with a balloon. The end-point of CAVEAT was restenosis rate and early results have shown a benefit for atherectomy (48 per cent versus 57 per cent). But the study sample was small ($n = 1012$), the end-point is impossible to judge from a clinical point of view, and the follow-up was short (6 months). The excitement generated by these studies of expensive and probably cost-ineffective technologies is out of all proportion to their real value to the patient at risk of coronary heart disease.

We have tried to show the clinical importance of intervention in five simple but pre-eminent factors which can bring about substantial reductions in cardiovascular morbidity and mortality. We believe that there is a need for a new way of managing patients with or at risk of coronary artery disease (CAD). To this end, we suggest the phrase 'cardioprotective therapeutics' to underline this new concept. Cardioprotective therapeutics straddles various specialties: cardiology, angiology, lipidology, clinical pharmacology and gynaecology. None of these taken alone adequately covers the single broad category of cardioprotection. If the long-term management of patients with (subclinical) CAD is to succeed in preventing further episodes of major cardiac decline, this integrated and holistic approach is essential. We believe that the checklist that our pentagon of protection brings to mind will be a helpful addition to the management of the complex influences in the course of ischaemic heart disease.

How is the field of cardioprotective therapeutics likely to develop?

# ■ EVOLVING THERAPY

Several large trials are in progress, each of which will shed further light on cardioprotective drug efficacy. For example, in the

Hypertension Optimal Treatment Study (HOT),[2] two key issues are under investigation. First, although we know that a difference in diastolic blood pressure of only 5–6 mmHg produces a 21 per cent reduction in cardiovascular mortality,[3] what is the optimum target diastolic blood pressure that should be achieved? This question is particularly important in the light of the debate over the J-shaped curve, in which risk is said to rise if blood pressure is lowered too far.[4] Thus, participants in the HOT trial will be randomized to one of three categories, aiming for a diastolic pressure of <90 mmHg, <85 mmHg, or <80 mmHg. Second, and of special interest in our discussion of an integrated approach to cardioprotection, patients will also be randomized within each of these diastolic blood pressure categories to either low-dose aspirin (75 mg/day) or placebo. A stepped-care approach to antihypertensive treatment is being applied, beginning with a calcium antagonist – felodipine – and subsequently adding a beta-blocker and an ACE inhibitor. About 18 000 hypertensive men and women will be enrolled and the first results are expected in 1996.

In other therapeutic areas, the Thrombosis Prevention Trial will examine the benefits of low-intensity oral anticoagulation with warfarin in men at risk of coronary heart disease;[5] head-to-head comparisons of statins and fibrates are likely; and, since GUSTO has shown differences between thrombolytic agents, new and more selective thrombolytic drugs will be developed.[6] Antiarrhythmic drugs will be designed which are more specifically directed at the processes leading to arrhythmogenesis in the ischaemic heart. Finally, the pressure for prospective studies of hormone replacement therapy with cardiovascular end-points will hopefully generate reliable data on which to base recommendations for women during the next 5–10 years. Although these refinements to our existing knowledge will be important, there is a law of diminishing returns from new clinical trials. We already know what key therapies work; this knowledge needs to be applied more widely.

Apart from testing new drugs in large trials, we will also target groups of patients at greater risk of coronary events. However, risk stratification has been discussed for several years, without much progress towards practicable clinical guidelines. A recent study illustrates the difficulties with this theoretically appealing idea.[7]

A substantial proportion of episodes of myocardial ischaemia are silent, i.e. symptom-free. Moss and his colleagues supposed that identification of these cases, together with those describing typical anginal symptoms, would be a powerful means of defining a high-risk group for aggressive treatment. Nine hundred and thirty-six patients who were judged to be clinically stable 1–6 months after an acute myocardial infarction (MI) were tested by rest, ambulatory and exercise electrocardiograms and stress thallium-201 scintigraphy. The only non-invasive variable that was associated with an increased risk of cardiac death, recurrent infarction or unstable angina during a 23-month follow-up was ST-segment depression on the resting ECG. An increased risk was also found when exercise-induced ST depression was present in association with diminished exercise duration or when reversible thallium defects were noted in patients who had increased pulmonary uptake. Each high-risk group made up only 3 per cent of the population under study. Thus, non-invasive methods of risk stratification seem to be insensitive tools for targeted treatment. More detailed assessment of the extent of coronary disease by coronary angiography might be necessary after all.

During the next 5 years, cardioprotective therapeutics will undergo fundamental changes in both its emphasis (earlier prevention) and direction (cellular and molecular targets).

# ■ DISCOVERING THE NEW

## □ Molecular genetics

Molecular genetic approaches to cardiovascular medicine are giving powerful insights into the factors that affect coronary risk and the treatments that are most likely to be effective.

Cambien and colleagues have shown that a deletion polymorphism in the gene encoding angiotensin-converting enzyme (ACE) is a risk factor for MI.[8] Circulating ACE concentrations are largely (about 50 per cent) determined genetically by an insertion (I)/deletion (D) polymorphism found on intron 16 of the ACE gene. The DD genotype is associated with higher concentrations of ACE than either the ID or II genotype. DD was significantly more common in 610 patients with an MI than in 733 controls. Furthermore, in a low-risk group (low plasma apo B concentrations, no lipid-lowering therapy, and low average body-mass index), the association of ACE/DD with myocardial infarction was significant across four geographically separate populations in Belfast, Lille, Strasbourg and Toulouse (Table 7.1). The overall population frequency of the ACE/DD genotype is 27 per cent. Thus, the total percentage of cases that might be attributable to this genotype is 8 per cent; in the low-risk group, the figure might be as high as 35 per cent. Given that about one-third to one-half of patients who have an MI have no identifiable conventional risk factors for CAD, this genetic marker is a potentially very important discovery. The same authors have also reported that the DD genotype is associated with a parental history of MI.[9] Do these findings provide a genetic link between hypertension and CAD?

Laboratory animal studies have shown that oestrogen influences the expression of kininogen genes that code for precursors of a family of vasoactive kinins.[10] Hepatic kininogen mRNA levels in female rats are four times higher than in their male counterparts. Oophorectomy decreases kininogen gene expression while oestrogen replacement increases kininogen mRNA levels. Serum immunoreactive kininogen is similarly influenced by oestrogen. Is this effect of a hormone on gene transcription the means by which oestrogen is cardioprotective? More generally, might gene manipulation be a key part of the future of cardioprotective therapeutics?

Some observers have urged caution on this question,[11] but there can be little doubt that the discovery of genetic susceptibility markers is likely to become an important component of population screening and risk stratification in the future.

One area of genetic research has yielded beneficial effects of gene therapy already. In a woman with familial hypercholesterolaemia, 10 per cent of her liver was removed, her hepatocytes were cultured in vitro, and these were then infected with a retrovirus vector containing the LDL receptor gene. These 'repaired' cells were infused back into the portal vein. The patient's LDL cholesterol was as high as 16.8 mmol/l before this procedure, but it has since fallen by up to 40 per cent without the addition of any lipid-lowering agent.[12] Analysis of liver biopsy samples has confirmed that the gene is working. Other transfection vectors – adenovirus and a 'pseudovirus' – are being tested and more patients are being recruited into these early gene therapy trials.

| | Belfast | | Lille | | Strasbourg | | Toulouse | | Total | |
|---|---|---|---|---|---|---|---|---|---|---|
| | Cases | Controls | Cases | Controls | Cases | Controls | Cases | Controls | Cases | Controls |
| **Low-risk group** | | | | | | | | | | |
| DD | 13 | 12 | 5 | 11 | 10 | 7 | 10 | 16 | 38 | 46 |
| ID+II | 15 | 40 | 1 | 28 | 14 | 28 | 11 | 47 | 41 | 143 |
| Odds ratio | 2.9(1.0–8.7) | | 12.7 | | 2.9(0.8–10.7) | | 2.7(0.8–8.4) | | 3.2(1.7–5.9) | |
| **High-risk group** | | | | | | | | | | |
| DD | 38 | 31 | 22 | 32 | 57 | 48 | 42 | 43 | 159 | 154 |
| ID+II | 135 | 97 | 30 | 77 | 123 | 111 | 84 | 105 | 372 | 390 |
| Odds ratio | 0.9(0.5–1.6) | | 1.8(0.8–3.7) | | 1.1(0.7–1.7) | | 1.2(0.7–2.1) | | 1.1(0.9–1.5) | |

Low-risk group: plasma apo B < 125 mg/dl; no hypolipidaemic drug treatment; body mass index < 26 <kg/m$^2$.

**Table 7.1** ACE genotypes according to risk status.

# ☐ Metabolic factors

As we come to understand the intracellular mechanisms of MI, we will be able to design drugs to intervene specifically in the processes either leading to or preventing ischaemic damage.

Cell damage leads to a cascade of adverse metabolic consequences (Figure 7.1)[13,14] that lead to left ventricular dysfunction and cell necrosis. Short episodes of myocardial ischaemia are associated with temporary myocardial dysfunction that gradually normalizes: the phenomenon of myocardial stunning.[15] Functional recovery may take several days. Once known, the biochemical factors associated with stunning should enable us to understand which processes allow ischaemic damage to be *reversible*. Re-establishing normal perfusion after temporary coronary occlusion leads to production of reactive oxygen species and lipid peroxides because of a dramatic rise in tissue oxygen (as superoxide). Electron transfer to these free radicals depends on several enzymes: xanthine oxidase, NADPH-cytochrome P450 reductase and cytochrome P450. Superoxide can be converted to

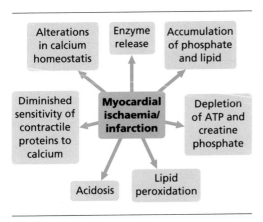

**Figure 7.1**
Metabolic influences of myocardial ischaemia/infarction.

$H_2O_2$ (by superoxide dismutase) and then, via glutathione peroxidase and catalase, to $H_2O_2$. Residual $H_2O_2$ can yield hydroxyl radicals that are especially damaging. Most of these processes take place in mitochondria, organelles that are particularly vulnerable to these reactive species.[16] Lipid peroxidation also takes place in mitochondria through $NADH-Fe^{3+}-ADP$-dependent processes.[17] Lipid peroxy radicals initiate widespread membrane lipid damage and eventually cell death. Many of these deleterious processes operate through changes in calcium flux. Increasing cytosolic calcium activates several enzymes – phospholipase $A_2$, proteases and endonucleases – that all have damaging effects on the cell.[18] Mitochondria, calcium and several key enzymes could clearly act as targets for new drugs.

## ☐ Ischaemic preconditioning

Ischaemic preconditioning is a recently reported phenomenon that seems to have powerful cardioprotective effects. Repetitive episodes of ischaemia with intervals of reperfusion can significantly limit subsequent infarction size.[19] Preliminary experiments in patients undergoing cardiopulmonary bypass in whom 3-min periods of aortic cross-clamping were followed by 2 min of reperfusion produced beneficial effects on myocardial enzyme leakage and ATP concentrations.[20] This process is probably mediated through adenosine.[21] From a clinical perspective, some intriguing data suggest that preconditioning may be occurring naturally in patients. Muller and colleagues[22] reported that subjects who had unstable angina before an MI had a better outcome postinfarction than other groups, although the former had a worse outlook in terms of coronary risk factors.

## ■ GETTING THE CONTEXT RIGHT

The benefits that can be achieved by drug therapy, together with the exciting prospects of genetic and metabolic manipulations, should not obscure the gains from two other very simple behavioural changes: stopping smoking and increasing exercise.

In a provocative analysis of the benefits to be gained by risk factor intervention, Yudkin has shown that stopping smoking in men will reduce their 10-year mortality from coronary heart disease (currently at around 14.4 per 1000) by 2.74 per 1000.[23] The corresponding figures for antihypertensive treatment, cholesterol lowering, and taking aspirin were 0.58, 0.82 and 2.64, respectively. These gains are even larger among men with diabetes (20.84 per 1000 for those stopping smoking). Yudkin calculated that between 2400 and 3800 man-years of drug treatment would be required to prevent one death from CAD in a non-diabetic man. Rates of morbidity from progression to angina or non-fatal MI were not taken into account. Such a startling statistic as this should neither obscure the fact that drug treatment *does* save lives nor ignore the importance of both the combined benefit of *multiple* risk factor intervention and targeting (perhaps genetically) particular at-risk groups. Nevertheless, the doctor should be aware of the quantitative benefits of such a simple behavioural modification.

In terms of our pentagon of protection, exercise has the capacity to reduce both systolic and diastolic blood pressure,[24] increase HDL and reduce LDL plasma concentrations,[25] and diminish the risk of thromboembolic complications.[26] Lack of exercise may be quantitatively as important as smoking, hypertension and hypercholesterolaemia.[27]

Overall lifestyle is important in all aspects of intervention. For instance, the Treatment of Mild Hypertension Study (TOMHS)[28] showed that patients who lose weight, become more active, drink less alcohol and eat less salt had substantial reductions in blood pressure on drug treatment (mean reduction of 16 mmHg in systolic blood pressure and 12 mmHg in diastolic pressure). Drug treatment *combined* with lifestyle alterations is a highly effective therapeutic regimen. Stress is also implicated in hypertension[29] and atherosclerosis[30] in laboratory animals and should be sought by the clinician who wishes to offer a complete programme of cardioprotective care.

Our approach to cardioprotective therapeutics has focused on drugs, but genetic, occupational and social factors all operate to influence the atherosclerotic disease process. We hope that our integrated vision of cardioprotection will overcome the boundaries created by different specialties and emerging fashions. We have an optimistic view of the future.

# References

1. Goldsmith MK, Revascularisation still the goal, strategy differs as cardiologists consider clinical trial results, *JAMA* (1993) **269**:450–1.

2. Hansson L, The Hypertension Optimal Treatment Study, *Blood Pressure* (1993) **2**:62–8.

3. Collins R, Peto R, MacMahon M et al, Blood pressure, stroke, and coronary heart-disease. Part 2, short-term reductions in blood pressure: overview of randomised drug trials in their epidemiological context, *Lancet* (1990) **335**:827–38.

4. Alderman MH, Ooi WL, Madharan S, Cohen H, Treatment-induced blood pressure reduction and the risk of myocardial infarction, *JAMA* (1989) **262**:920–4.

5. Meade TW, Roderick PJ, Bremnan PJ et al, Extracranial bleeding and other symptoms due to low-dose aspirin and low-intensity oral anti-coagulation, *Thromb Haemost* (1992) **68**:1–6.

6. Collen D, Towards improved thrombolytic therapy, *Lancet* (1993) **342**: 34–6.

7. Moss AJ, Goldstein RE, Hall J et al, Detection and significance of myocardial ischaemia in stable patients after recovery from an acute coronary event, *JAMA* (1993) **269**:2379–85.

8. Cambian F, Poirier O, Lecerf L et al, Deletion polymorphism in the gene for angiotensin-converting enzyme is a potent risk factor for myocardial infarction, *Nature* (1992) **359**:641–4.

9 Tiret L, Kee F, Poirier O et al, Deletion polymorphism in angiotensin-converting enzyme gene associated with parental history of myocardial infarction, *Lancet* (1993) **341**:991–2.

10 Chen LM, Chung P, Chao S, Chao L, Chao J, Differential regulation of kininogen gene expression by estrogen and progesterone in vivo, *Biochim Biophys Acta* (1992) **1131**:145–51.

11. Swales JD, The ACE gene: a cardiovascular risk factor, *J R Coll Phys* (1993) **27**:106–8.

12. Randall T, First gene therapy for inherited hypercholesterolaemia a partial success, *JAMA* (1993) **269**:837–8.

13. Orrenius S, McConkey DJ, Bellomo G, Nicotera P, Role of calcium in toxic cell killing, *Trends Pharmacol Sci* (1989) **10**:281–5.

14. Gauduel U, Menasche P, Durelleroy M, Enzyme release and mitochondrial activity in reoxygenated cardiac muscle: relationship with oxygen-induced lipid peroxidation, *Gen Physiol Biophys* (1989) **8**:327–40.

15. Braunwald E, Kloner RA, The stunned myocardium-prolonged post-ischemic ventricular dysfunction, *Circulation* (1982) **66**:1146–9.

16. Hruszkewycz AM, Bergtold DS. Oxygen radicals, lipid peroxidation, and DNA damage in mitochondria, *Basic Life Sci* (1988) **49**:449–56.

17. Bindoli A, Lipid peroxidation in mitochondria, *Free Radic Biol Med* (1988) **5**:247–61.

18. Nicotera P, McConkey DJ, Dypbukt JM, Jones DP, Orrenius S, Calcium activated mechanisms in cell killing, *Drug Metab Rev* (1989) **20**:193–201.

19. Walker DM, Yellon DM, Ischaemic preconditioning: from mechanisms to exploitation, *Cardiovasc Res* (1992) **26**:734–9.

20. Yellon DM, Walker JM, Klorer RA, Downey JM, Pugsley WB, Unstable angina, *Lancet* (1993) **351**:1223–7.

21. Liu GS, Thornton J, Van Winkle DM et al, Protection against infarction afforded by preconditioning is mediated by A1 adenosine receptors in rabbit heart, *Circulation* (1991) **84**:350–6.

22. Muller DW, Topoi EJ, Califf RM et al, Relation between antecedent angina pectoris and short-term prognosis after thrombolytic therapy for acute myocardial infarction, *Am Heart J* (1990) **119**:224–31.

23. Yudkin JS. How can we best prolong life? Benefits of coronary risk factor reduction in non–diabetic and diabetic subjects, *Br Med J* (1993) **306**:1313–18.

24. Nelson L, Jennings GL, Ecler MD, Komer PI, Effect of changing levels of physical inactivity on blood pressure and haemodynamics in essential hypertension, *Lancet* (1986) **ii**:473–6.

25. Hardman AE, Hudson J, Jones PRM, Norgan NG, Brisk walking and high density lipoprotein cholesterol concentration in formerly sedentary women.*Br Med J* (1989) **299**:1204–5.

26. Ferguson EW, Bernier LL, Barton GR, Yu-Yehiro J, Schoomaker EB, Effects of exercise and conditioning on clotting and fibrinolytic activity in men, *J Appl Physiol* (1987) **62**:1416–21.

27. Powell KE, Thompson PD, Casperson CJ, Kendrick JS, Physical activity and the incidence of coronary heart disease, *Ann Rev Public Health* (1987) **8**:253–87.

28. Goldsmith MF, Treatment of mild hypertension study shows results better when drugs abet lifestyle changes, *JAMA* (1993) **269**:323–4.

29. Henry JP, Ely DL, Stephens PM et al, The role of psychosocial factors in the development of arteriosclerosis in CBA mice, *Atherosclerosis* (1971) **14**:203–6.

30 Kaplan JR, Manuck SB, Clarkson TB, Lusso FM, Taub DM, Social status, environment, and atherosclerosis in cynomolgus monkeys, *Arteriosclerosis* (1982) **2**:359–64.

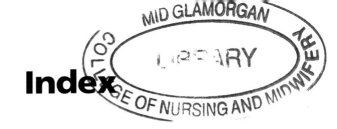

# Index

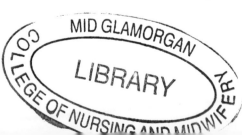